Hepatitis C

A Hazelden Pocket Health Guide

Hepatitis C

*Practical, Medical, and Spiritual
Guidelines for Daily Living with HCV*

MARK JENKINS

Foreword by Robert E. Larsen, M.D.

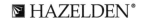
INFORMATION & EDUCATIONAL SERVICES

Hazelden
Center City, Minnesota 55012-0176

1-800-328-0094
1-651-213-4590 (Fax)
www.hazelden.org

Library of Congress Cataloging-in-Publication Data

Jenkins, Mark, 1962–
    Hepatitis C : practical, medical, and spiritual guidelines for daily living
    with HCV / Mark Jenkins ; foreword by Robert E. Larsen.
        p. cm. — (A Hazelden pocket health guide)
    Includes bibliographical references and index.
    ISBN 1-56838-368-1
    1. Hepatitis C—Popular works. 2. Twelve-step programs. 3. Hepatitis
C—Psychological aspects. 4. Hepatitis C—Social aspects. 5. Adjustment
(Pychology) I. Title. II. Series.

RC848.H425 J46 2000
362.1'963623—dc21   99-058532

04 03 02 01 00   6 5 4 3 2

Editor's note
The excerpt from the text *Alcoholics Anonymous,* pages 83–84, and the
Twelve Steps of Alcoholics Anonymous are reprinted and adapted with permission of Alcoholics Anonymous World Services, Inc (AAWS). Permission
to reprint and adapt the Twelve Steps does not mean that AAWS has reviewed
or approved the contents of this publication, or that AAWS necessarily agrees
with the views expressed herein. AA is a program of recovery from alcoholism *only*—use of this excerpt and the Twelve Steps in connection with programs and activities which are patterned after AA, but which address other
problems, or in any other non-AA context, does not imply otherwise.

Cover design by David Spohn
Interior design by Donna Burch
Typesetting by Stanton Publication Services, Inc.

Contents

Foreword

For the past sixty years, millions of addicts and alcoholics have stopped using drugs and found new, rewarding lives by following the spiritual principles outlined in Twelve Step programs such as Alcoholics Anonymous. From a medical perspective, it is not unreasonable to say that Twelve Step programs constitute the gold standard of treatment for the chronic disease of chemical dependency. These programs have been so successful that they are now used to deal with other challenges of a chronic nature, such as overeating, sexual compulsion, gambling, and depression.

The Hazelden Pocket Health Guide series is designed to help patients cope with chronic diseases, specifically, diseases that may be the result of an addiction. These long-term, potentially debilitating illnesses include chronic obstructive pulmonary disease (COPD), hypertension, HIV/AIDS, and liver disease. This series can help patients use the same spiritual principles that have enabled so many chemically dependent people to lead full and satisfying lives.

Spirituality and acceptance are powerful tools patients and health care professionals can apply to help deal with disease. In thirty years of medical practice, I have seen many patients with chronic disease who, despite the best physicians and hospitals, have done poorly. Sometimes this was due to the severity of the disease process, but often, the patient's inability to accept the disease and its consequences was significant. Denial is a common problem in chemically dependent people, but chemical dependency is by no means the only disease in which it plays a major role in the outcome. Denial is common to *every* chronic disease known to medical science. If not dealt with effectively, it is a major stumbling block to effective treatment.

Despite significant advances in treating diabetes, for instance, at least half of all diabetics fail to follow their diets or to take their medications properly. Many of these patients suffer amputations, kidney failure and dialysis, heart attacks, and blindness partly due to their disease but mostly due to the denial that blinds them to effective treatment of the disease.

Denial and chronic disease can be dealt with by using spiritual principles. Spirituality is not religion, although some people achieve it in traditional religious communities. Spirituality is the concept that each of us has a Higher Power that can help us cope with life. For many this is the traditional God, while for others it may be nature, the recovering community, or a set of guiding principles. Each person has his or her own concept of a Higher Power. Spirituality is not a particular religious dogma but rather a concept that allows people to feel good about how they live their lives.

Bill Wilson, the cofounder of Alcoholics Anonymous, described spirituality as the concept that we can do together what we could not do alone. Spirituality is about community and being a part of a greater whole. Spirituality is we *not* me.

Hepatitis C

Hepatitis C, the quiet epidemic. Fifteen years ago, medical science was not aware of this disease. Now experts say the death rate from hepatitis C will triple over the next ten to twenty years. Hepatitis C (or HCV) is a viral disease. As with most viral illnesses, the body forms antibodies against it. HCV, however, is different because in 80 percent of cases the antibodies that are formed do not protect the patient from progression of the disease. For the vast majority, HCV is a lifelong disease. Fortunately, for most patients, it produces only minor symptoms. Unfortunately, about 20 percent of HCV-positive people die from cirrhosis of the liver or cancer of the liver. While HCV can be treated to some degree, it cannot be cured using today's technology. HCV sufferers must learn how to cope, while they let medical science do what it can.

A wise old professor of medicine once said, "Disease is what you have and illness is how you react to it." It is possible to see patients who have severe disease with minimal illness. Still others have mild disease but severe illness. As with all forms of chronic disease, the secret to dealing with the situation is in the patient's reaction to his or her disease. You cannot be cured, but you can exert considerable influence over this disease.

We wish you well on your journey.

Robert E. Larsen, M.D.
Coordinator, Health Care Professionals Program
Hazelden Foundation

Preface

I owe my life to a spiritual program of recovery. My journey started when I joined the recovery community. By following the Twelve Steps of Alcoholics Anonymous (AA) (the basis of all Twelve Step programs), I found a new life. My career was rebuilt, my relationships with others mended, my self-esteem restored.

A natural-born cynic, I was at first astounded when so many of "the Promises" I had been told about came true, and in such short order (see pages xix–xx for more on the Promises). Even by then, I had learned not to question but simply to accept such blessings as part of my continuing journey.

As a medical writer with several books to my credit, I began to postulate that this spiritual program of recovery would be a revelation to people with chronic illnesses. After all, the Twelve Steps are a universal plan for living well. Countless groups apply the Twelve Steps to their addictions and conditions, including Emotions Anonymous, Debtors Anonymous, Gamblers Anonymous, and, the grandparent of them all, Alcoholics Anonymous. And so I set about writing a book that offers a spiritual program of recovery from chronic illness.

Probably no one needs a guide to living well more

than people who suffer from a long-term medical condition. Chronic illness affects more than ninety million Americans and, according to the American Medical Association, is the nation's foremost health concern. Chronic illness can lead to feelings of anger, isolation, and loneliness, financial difficulties, compromised personal relationships, and trouble at work. The emotional consequences of a chronic illness are especially profound when the condition is caused by a dependency on a mood-altering substance such as nicotine or alcohol. The Twelve Step program helps people deal with these emotions by teaching them how to find their spirituality.

I am hardly the first person to suggest that the Twelve Steps can benefit those with chronic illnesses. Many others whose lives have been transformed by a Twelve Step program have applied these principles to conditions ranging from cancer to AIDS. For the person with a specific chronic illness, however, what has been lacking in these interpretations is a plan for individual conditions. Until now.

This book is part of the Hazelden Pocket Health Guide series, a series of books that adapts the Twelve Steps for those with chronic illnesses—in this case, hepatitis C (HCV for short). The book combines specific medical guidelines with a plan to improve emotional and spiritual well-being. At its core is a program of hope, happiness, and healing.

Above all, this program gives those with chronic illnesses such as HCV what they need: the indispensable tools and inspiration to live life one day at a time—and to live it well.

Spirituality: The Strongest Medicine of All?

Can spirituality help me beat my disease? That's probably the question you're asking yourself. A better question might be, Can the spiritual program this book teaches help me manage my disease more effectively? The answer to that question is "yes."

The National Institutes of Health recognizes spirituality as an important component of alternative and complementary medicine. No wonder. A growing body of evidence suggests that spirituality actually helps people stay healthy and recover from illness.

In one of the most extensive laboratory studies ever done on the subject of spirituality and disease, researchers at Harvard's Mind/Body Medical Institute recently found that prayer and meditation—prerequisites for a sound spiritual life—cause a person's body to undergo healthful changes.[1] Metabolism, heart rate, and rate of breathing decrease, and brain waves slow down. These changes are the opposite of those induced

---

1. For a brochure describing the Mind/Body Medical Institute, call (617) 632-9525 or visit its Web site at www.mindbody.harvard.edu

by stress and are an effective therapy for certain diseases, especially those chronic in nature. Significantly, many doctors believe that because stress worsens a disease, a spiritual program that involves prayer and meditation is an effective component of treatment. If this is true, it is only logical to conclude that spirituality benefits those who have hepatitis C (HCV).

Although skeptics still question whether the chronically ill person who is spiritual is more likely to benefit medically than someone who is not spiritual, of this there is no doubt: spirituality helps chronically ill people cope with the emotional challenges of their condition.

But just what is spirituality, anyway? One thing it isn't is religion. Although many truly religious people are spiritual, and many spiritual people consider themselves to be religious, the two concepts are not one and the same. A person doesn't have to be religious to be spiritual. Religion is a formalization of society's relationship with God into rituals and institutions. Spirituality is an inherent belief in the existence of a Higher Power, energy, or force—one that a person may or may not choose to call God—and a feeling of closeness to that entity. That being is referred to variously within these pages as a Higher Power, a Power greater than ourselves, or a Power Greater.

This book advocates use of the Twelve Steps, a

spiritual program founded in the 1930s to help alcoholics recover from the disease of alcoholism. The
Twelve Steps can help you "turn over" care of your
disease to a Higher Power that is greater and wiser
than you, and that loves you. The program will help
you maintain strength and hope as you live each day
with your disease.

You'll learn in depth about the Twelve Steps later
in this book. Right now what's important is that you
know that managing HCV isn't just about arresting the
medical aspects of the disease, although you will certainly learn most of what you need to know in these
pages. No, managing HCV is also about living well
with that chronic illness every day.

The Twelve Steps will help you do this by allowing you to recognize what you do and don't have control over. In cooperation with your Higher Power, you
have the wisdom to deal with your feelings about your
disease and to change the behaviors that caused the
condition, as well as to take certain steps to prevent it
from getting worse, such as exercising, abstaining
from alcohol, and taking your medication. The Twelve
Steps will also show you how to grow spiritually
through prayer, meditation, and support.

Currently there is no known cure for HCV, just as
there is no cure for alcoholism and other chronic illnesses. If you practice the principles outlined in the

Twelve Steps, however, they will improve your ability to accept and live with your disease, and will offer you a way of life you may never have experienced had you not been stricken with a chronic illness.

Despite their popularity, Twelve Step programs are still widely misunderstood in some quarters. Such misunderstandings stand in the way of their acceptance by those who could really use them, including people with chronic illnesses such as HCV. Perhaps the most common misunderstanding is that Twelve Step programs are "covers" for religion and, specifically, Christian groups.

A hasty reading of the Steps may reinforce this impression; however, reading more carefully you'll discover that the Steps do not endorse any religion. A person who lives by the Steps could be Jewish, Christian, Hindu, Muslim, Buddhist, agnostic, or atheist.

If the Twelve Steps are not a religious program, then they certainly are a spiritual one. The Steps echo what writer Aldous Huxley called the "perennial philosophy"—a core set of ideas and practices shared by many religious traditions. The Steps have one major concern and that is human transformation.

You may already be intimately familiar with a Twelve Step program. If you have not experienced the Steps, you will discover that they offer a new approach to living. This approach is available to you if you acknowledge your jeopardy and your need to change your behaviors and to improve your state of being.

The spiritual component of this book draws extensively on principles developed by the founders of Alcoholics Anonymous. Like alcoholism, HCV is a chronic disease. And as with alcoholics, if you don't do what's necessary to address your condition, your disease will come to profoundly affect your life and to eventually kill you.

Alcoholics must abstain from alcohol and other drugs. As a person with HCV, you must follow a strict drug regimen, abstain from alcohol, and get vaccinated against other forms of hepatitis. The extraordinary success achieved by millions of participants in Twelve Step programs who now abstain from alcohol and other drugs can be emulated by those with HCV who follow the Steps suggested in this book.

It is heartening to know that the Promises that inspire Alcoholics Anonymous members also offer strength and hope to people with HCV who are willing to follow this simple program:

> If we are painstaking about this phase of our development, we will be amazed before we are half way through. We are going to know a new freedom and a new happiness. We will not regret the past nor wish to shut the door on it. We will

comprehend the word serenity and we will know peace. No matter how far down the scale we have gone, we will see how our experience can benefit others. That feeling of uselessness and self-pity will disappear. We will lose interest in selfish things and gain interest in our fellows. Self-seeking will slip away. Our whole attitude and outlook upon life will change. Fear of people and of economic insecurity will leave us. We will intuitively know how to handle situations which used to baffle us. We will suddenly realize that God is doing for us what we could not do for ourselves.[2]

The Twelve Step program of spirituality discussed in this book stresses acceptance. Only when you accept that you have HCV and that it can be the cause of serious health consequences will you be able to take the steps necessary to address the disease. Not only will denial prevent you from addressing the spiritual component of your chronic disease but also in a very real way it will delay you from taking the vital medical measures necessary to improve and extend your life. Thus, the first part of this book describes the chronic disease of HCV, its symptoms, causes, and treatment.

---

2. *Alcoholics Anonymous,* 3d ed. (New York: Alcoholics Anonymous World Services, Inc., 1976), 83–84. Reprinted with permission.

The Twelve Steps for Hepatitis C[3]

Step One—We admitted we were powerless over chronic illness—that our lives had become unmanageable.

Step Two—Came to believe that a Power greater than ourselves could restore us to sanity.

Step Three—Made a decision to turn our will and our lives over to the care of a Power greater than ourselves.

Step Four—Made a searching and fearless moral inventory of ourselves.

Step Five—Admitted to the God of our understanding, to ourselves, and to another human being the exact nature of our wrongs.

Step Six—Were entirely ready to have the God of our understanding remove all these defects of character.

Step Seven—Humbly asked our Higher Power to remove our shortcomings.

Step Eight—Made a list of all persons we had harmed, and became willing to make amends to them all.

Step Nine—Made direct amends to such people wherever possible, except when to do so would injure them or others.

3. Adapted from the Twelve Steps of Alcoholics Anonymous with the permission of AA World Services, Inc., New York, N.Y.

Step Ten—Continued to take personal inventory and when we were wrong promptly admitted it.

Step Eleven—Sought through prayer and meditation to improve our conscious contact with a Power greater than ourselves, praying only for knowledge of our Higher Power's will and the courage to carry that out.

Step Twelve—Having had a spiritual awakening as the result of these Steps, we tried to carry our message to others with our condition and to practice these principles in all our affairs.

The Twelve Steps of Alcoholics Anonymous[4]

Step One—We admitted we were powerless over alcohol—that our lives had become unmanageable.

Step Two—Came to believe that a Power greater than ourselves could restore us to sanity.

Step Three—Made a decision to turn our will and our lives over to the care of God *as we understood Him.*

Step Four—Made a searching and fearless moral inventory of ourselves.

Step Five—Admitted to God, to ourselves, and

4. The Twelve Steps of AA are taken from *Alcoholics Anonymous,* 3d ed., published by AA World Services, Inc., New York, N.Y., 59–60. Reprinted with permission of AA World Services, Inc. (See editor's note on copyright page.)

to another human being the exact nature of our wrongs.

Step Six—Were entirely ready to have God remove all these defects of character.

Step Seven—Humbly asked Him to remove our shortcomings.

Step Eight—Made a list of all persons we had harmed, and became willing to make amends to them all.

Step Nine—Made direct amends to such people wherever possible, except when to do so would injure them or others.

Step Ten—Continued to take personal inventory and when we were wrong promptly admitted it.

Step Eleven—Sought through prayer and meditation to improve our conscious contact with God *as we understood Him,* praying only for knowledge of His will for us and the power to carry that out.

Step Twelve—Having had a spiritual awakening as the result of these steps, we tried to carry this message to alcoholics, and to practice these principles in all our affairs.

CHAPTER ONE

Hepatitis C Essentials

During the 1970s, medical scientists became aware of the spread of an aggressive virus that attacked the liver. The disease affected the body in much the same way that known forms of the hepatitis virus (A and B) did. Chiefly, this new virus caused liver inflammation, but unlike patients who contracted hepatitis A and hepatitis B, those who were diagnosed with this new virus couldn't get rid of it. Its defining characteristic was that in most patients it tenaciously stayed in their bodies and continued to go on damaging their livers, eventually causing death. Because tests showed that these patients had neither hepatitis A nor B, doctors dubbed the condition "non-A, non-B hepatitis."

Finally, in 1989, doctors identified the cause of the mysterious liver disease. It was a virulent strain of hepatitis they called the hepatitis C virus, HCV for short.

Since its discovery over twenty years ago, HCV has become a leading public health concern in the United

States and an even more widespread medical crisis worldwide.

Unlike other forms of hepatitis, HCV is difficult for the immune system to overcome, and so the disease can cause serious, long-term liver damage, including cirrhosis, liver cancer, and even liver failure—all three of which can be fatal. Among those who contract acute HCV, 85 percent develop a chronic form of the disease, 70 percent develop symptoms such as fatigue and joint aches, 15 percent develop cirrhosis, and 5 percent die as a result of chronic liver disease such as cancer or cirrhosis.

Fortunately, though, the disease usually progresses slowly. It can be between ten and forty years before symptoms are first felt. Also, when it's caught early, treatment and lifestyle changes can stop or slow down the disease's progression. Many people outlive the virus, dying from other causes before HCV becomes a problem.

It is estimated that four million Americans have HCV. The virus is especially prevalent among minorities—studies show that 3.2 percent of African Americans and 2.1 percent of Mexican Americans have HCV. At present, HCV is responsible for up to ten thousand deaths a year in the United States. If the disease continues to spread unabated, that number will triple over the next ten to twenty years, eventually killing more people than AIDS kills. After alcohol-related cirrhosis, HCV is now the leading cause of liver transplants in the United States.

Chronic versus Acute HCV

This book is primarily for people with chronic HCV. However, it is important for readers to understand the difference between the terms "chronic" and "acute" hepatitis. Acute HCV is the initial infection phase. There may or may not be flulike symptoms associated with this phase. If detected and treated within six months, the virus may go away. If the virus goes undetected and untreated (as is what usually happens), or if it is diagnosed but treatment cannot rid the body of the virus, the condition becomes chronic. Even though there may be no symptoms, slow but inevitable damage to the liver takes place. The rate at which this liver damage occurs varies considerably; sometimes it is virtually undetectable for decades.

Given that symptoms of HCV are often not felt for decades after initial infection, and that a bulk of the infections took place as recently as the mid- to late-1980s, the true impact of this disease has yet to be felt.

As a result, little attention has been given to HCV,

causing some to call it the "silent epidemic." Because of the grave dangers associated with HCV, it is important to learn about this life-threatening virus—especially if you are at risk of contracting it or may already have it.

Early detection is especially important. Finding out early whether you have HCV can help you in the following ways:

- You can get medication, which, the sooner it starts, the more effective it will be.
- You can take tests to see how much liver damage has occurred.
- You can learn how to protect your liver from further damage through diet and lifestyle changes such as abstaining from alcohol.
- You can learn how to prevent transmitting the infection to others.

How Does Hepatitis C Progress?

Most acute HCV infections become chronic because the immune system cannot rid the body of the virus. The virus takes over more and more liver cells and keeps spreading. In this way a large number of liver cells become scarred and damaged. You may not feel any symptoms at all until so much damage has occurred that your liver won't function properly. This can take decades, depending on how aggressive the virus inside you is and how well you take care of your health.

The rate of progression for HCV is generally very slow. Under certain circumstances, however, the disease can progress rapidly leading to death from liver failure. Alcohol consumption is a frequent cause of a rapid progression of HCV. A person with HCV who drinks even a moderate amount of alcohol will put such a severe strain on the liver that rapid liver damage will inevitably occur. A frequent result is death.

How Is HCV Transmitted?

HCV is a blood-borne virus. To catch it you need to come into contact with infected blood. Blood transfusions are the most likely cause of HCV infection. Before 1990, authorities did not test donated blood for HCV (the disease was only identified in 1989), and the likelihood of infection was about 10 percent in people who had transfusions. Since HCV detection measures were introduced in the early 1990s, transmissions through the blood supply have dropped to virtually zero. Still, thousands of new cases of HCV are diagnosed each year. Today, it is estimated that 60 percent of new infections are through intravenous drug use and 20 percent through sexual activity. Other means of transmission include poorly sterilized medical instruments, blood spills, unbandaged cuts or injuries, and tattooing or piercing. It is also possible for expectant mothers with HCV to pass it on to their unborn children.

Who Is at Risk?

The following groups of people are at increased risk of HCV:

- recipients of blood transfusions before July 1992
- intravenous drug users
- hemodialysis patients
- recipients of blood-clotting factors made before 1987
- health care workers
- children born to infected mothers
- people who have had multiple sex partners

In about 10 percent of cases, it is impossible to determine how a person contracted HCV.

Protecting Yourself from Getting HCV

These recommendations on preventing HCV transmission are from the federal government's Centers for Disease Control:

- *Don't ever shoot drugs. If you do shoot drugs, stop and get into a treatment program. If you relapse, never reuse or share syringes, water, or drug works, and get vaccinated against hepatitis A and hepatitis B.*
- *Don't share toothbrushes, razors, or other personal-care articles. They may have blood on them.*

- *If you are a health care worker, always follow routine barrier precautions and safely handle needles and other sharp objects that may have blood on them. And get vaccinated against hepatitis B.*
- *Consider the health risks if you are thinking about getting a tattoo or body piercing. You can get infected if*
  - *the tools being used have someone else's blood on them*
  - *the artist or piercer doesn't observe healthy practices such as handwashing and using disposable gloves*

HCV can be spread through sex, although this does not occur very often. If you are sexually active with more than one partner, always use condoms.

What Are the Symptoms?

Most people who have early-stage HCV experience mild symptoms that may be indistinguishable from just feeling run-down. The most common symptom, which may not begin until years after the initial infection, is fatigue. Other symptoms are mild fever, joint and muscle aches, loss of appetite, nonspecific abdominal pain, occasional nausea, and sometimes diarrhea. Early on, many people with HCV dismiss the symptoms as a flu that comes and goes. As the disease progresses, different symptoms begin to be felt. These symptoms reflect damage to the liver as seen in people with cirrhosis and liver failure: jaundice, abdominal swelling (due to fluid retention called "ascites"), and finally, coma. It may take as long as forty years for these symptoms to develop. Sometimes they do not occur at all.

Primary Symptoms of HCV

Mental:

- *depression*
- *anger*
- *fear and anxiety*

Physical:

- *fatigue*
- *joint and muscle aches and pains*
- *headaches*
- *nausea and loss of appetite*

How Is HCV Diagnosed?

One of the goals of medical scientists who specialize in HCV is to find more effective ways to diagnose this disease. Tests to detect the virus are now very accurate, although it is not quite as easy to determine levels of the virus, whether the disease is acute or chronic, and how much damage has been done to the liver.

Often people who have HCV do not realize they have been infected because they do not have any symptoms. Only years later, and often only by chance, do they find out—when getting their blood tested to qualify for life insurance, getting a marriage license, undergoing fertility therapy, or donating blood.

In such cases a standard blood test called an ALT test may reveal liver inflammation, a possible sign of HCV infection. An ALT test measures the amount of the enzyme "alanine aminotransferase" (ALT) in your blood. An elevated ALT is a sign of liver inflammation. A positive ALT test demonstrates only that there is liver inflammation; it does not reveal what the cause is. Further tests are necessary to determine the cause of the inflammation (ALT tests may be used later to check your liver to see if your disease is worsening or if treatment is working).

To find out if HCV is causing the damage to your liver revealed by the ALT test, your doctor will have to do a test specifically to see whether the HCV virus or telltale antibodies are present in your blood. Several tests may be done. Each will tell you something different about your exposure to HCV.

Usually the first test done is an "enzyme immuno-assay test" (EIA) to test for antibodies to HCV. If the test detects the presence of HCV antibodies, then almost certainly the virus is present. EIA tests are between 90 and 95 percent accurate; however, even if it shows positive, the test doesn't reveal whether you have acute or chronic HCV—only that the virus is present in your blood.

To get more information, your doctor may order the "recombinant immunoblot assay test" (RIBA), another test to detect antibodies, or a "polymerase chain reaction test" (PCR) to establish how much of the virus is in your system. These tests are done only to confirm the diagnosis or to measure the progression of the disease.

The most accurate way to assess the extent of liver damage in a person who has HCV is with a liver biopsy. In this test a small piece of liver is removed and examined (the piece is too small to affect the function of your liver). Because a liver biopsy is a surgical procedure, and any invasive procedure involves a certain amount of risk, not to mention discomfort and expense, many doctors prefer nonsurgical means of testing—at least initially. Later on, a liver biopsy may be necessary to see whether your disease is worsening or whether treatment is slowing down its progress. If you already have obvious signs of advanced liver disease, a biopsy probably won't be necessary.

Can HCV Be Cured?

At present there is no cure for chronic HCV. By far, the most effective way to treat the virus is with long-term, aggressive drug therapy, but this works in less than half of patients. However, because HCV develops so slowly, even when drug therapy is not effective, people infected with HCV who make the appropriate changes in their lifestyles can usually enjoy long life expectancies and, just as important, lead healthy lives. Much more about drug treatment for HCV can be found in chapter 3.

Anatomy of the Hepatitis C Virus

Viruses are the smallest known forms of life. Their goal is to invade host cells—including human body cells—which they turn into tiny "factories" where they multiply. This process eventually kills the host cells, allowing the disease to develop.

Viruses are selective. They usually infect only one cell group such as the lungs (pneumonia) or liver (hepatitis). Different viruses, therefore, cause different diseases.

It is rare that viruses affect different species. Many diseases in humans are caused by viruses. Some, such as the flu or the common cold, can be relatively harmless, while others, including smallpox, AIDS, and hepatitis, are potentially deadly.

Humans have developed defenses against viruses—most important, the immune system, which can disarm and then destroy viruses. But when the immune system is weakened or overpowered, the disease cells take over.

HCV is an especially small virus. It is approximately fifty nanometers across (a nanometer is one billionth of a meter). If you placed two hundred thousand HCV side by side, they would only be one centimeter long.

Despite its size, HCV is extremely aggressive. It is a rare example of an RNA virus that foils the human immune system. RNA viruses do this by altering their structure—or mutating—in such a way that the immune system cannot adapt fast enough to fight them. Thus, more than 80 percent of people who contract acute HCV cannot get the virus out of their systems, and they develop chronic HCV. Unlike most epidemics, which kill a relatively small number of people before the population develops an immunity to the virus and it dies out, HCV stays a step ahead of the human immune system and of scientists trying to develop a cure.

The ABC's of Hepatitis

Hepatitis C is one of at least six forms of viral hepatitis that attack the liver: hepatitis A, B, C, D, E, and G. The following table provides basic information about the most common forms of hepatitis.[1]

---

1. Reproduced with permission from the Hepatitis Foundation International, 30 Sunrise Terrace, Cedar Grove, NJ 07009-1423; phone: (973) 239-1035 or (800) 891-0707; fax: (973) 857-5044; e-mail: mail@hepfi.org; Web site: www.hepfi.org

	Hepatitis A (HAV)	Hepatitis B (HBV)	Hepatitis C (HCV)	Hepatitis D (HDV)	Hepatitis E (HEV)
What is it?	HAV is a virus that causes inflammation of the liver. It does not lead to chronic disease.	HBV is a virus that causes inflammation of the liver. The virus can cause liver cell damage, leading to cirrhosis and cancer.	HCV is a virus that causes inflammation of the liver. This infection can lead to cirrhosis and cancer.	HDV is a virus that causes inflammation of the liver. It infects those persons with HBV.	HEV is a virus that causes inflammation of the liver. It is rare in the U.S. There is no chronic state.
Incubation period	2 to 7 weeks. Average 4 weeks.	6 to 23 weeks. Average 17 weeks.	2 to 25 weeks. Average 7 to 9 weeks.	2 to 8 weeks.	2 to 9 weeks. Average 6 weeks.
How is it spread?	Transmitted by fecal/oral route, through close person-to-person contact or ingestion of contaminated food and water.	Contact with infected blood, seminal fluid, vaginal secretions; contaminated drug needles, including tattoo/ body piercing tools. Infected mother to newborn. Human bite. Sexual contact.	Contact with infected blood; contaminated needles, razors, and tattoo or body piercing tools. Infected mother to newborn. NOT easily spread through sex.	Contact with infected blood, contaminated needles. Sexual contact with HDV-infected person.	Transmitted through fecal/oral route. Outbreaks associated with contaminated water supply in other countries.

	Hepatitis A (HAV)	Hepatitis B (HBV)	Hepatitis C (HCV)	Hepatitis D (HDV)	Hepatitis E (HEV)
Symptoms	May have none. Others may have light stools, dark urine, fatigue, fever, nausea, vomiting, abdominal pain, and jaundice.	May have none. Some persons have mild flu-like symptoms, dark urine, light stools, jaundice, fatigue, and fever.	Same as HBV.	Same as HBV.	Same as HBV.
Treatment of chronic disease	Not applicable.	Antiviral medications with varying success.	Interferon and combination therapies with varying success.	Interferon with varying success.	Not applicable.
Vaccine	Two doses of vaccine to anyone over 2 years of age.	Three doses may be given to persons of any age.	None.	HBV vaccine prevents HDV infection.	None.
Who is at risk?	Household or sexual contact with an infected person or living in an area with HAV outbreak. Travelers	Infant born to infected mother, having sex with infected person or multiple partners, injection drug users,	Blood transfusion recipients before July 1992, health care workers, injection drug users, hemodialysis patients,	Injection drug users, persons engaging in anal/oral sex, and those having sex with an HDV-infected person.	Travelers to developing countries, especially pregnant women.

	Hepatitis A (HAV)	Hepatitis B (HBV)	Hepatitis C (HCV)	Hepatitis D (HDV)	Hepatitis E (HEV)
	to developing countries, persons engaging in anal/oral sex, and injection drug users.	emergency responders, health care workers, persons engaging in anal/oral sex, and hemodialysis patients.	infants born to infected mother, multiple sex partners.		
Prevention	Immune Globulin within 2 weeks of exposure. Vaccination. Washing hands with soap and water after going to the toilet. Use household bleach to clean surfaces contaminated with feces, such as changing tables. Safe sex.	Immune Globulin within 2 weeks of exposure. Vaccination provides protection for 18 years. Clean up infected blood with household bleach and wear protective gloves. Do not share razors, toothbrushes, or needles. Safe sex.	Clean up spilled blood with household bleach. Wear protective gloves. Do not share razors, toothbrushes, or needles. Safe sex.	Hepatitis B vaccine to prevent HBV infection. Safe sex.	Avoid drinking or using potentially contaminated water.

Who Should Get Tested?

The sooner HCV is detected, the more quickly treatment can start. Treatment may slow the progression of the disease and minimize its harmful effects. Unfortunately, because symptoms may take decades to develop, most people don't know they have HCV until the disease has progressed to the stage where significant, life-threatening liver damage has already occurred.

All this reinforces the need for early diagnosis. You should definitely be tested for HCV if you answer yes to one or more of the following questions:

- Did you have a blood transfusion before 1992?
- Have you ever injected drugs into your body?
- Have you had a tattoo done on your body or had any part of your body pierced?
- Have you had multiple sex partners?
- Have you or your partner ever been treated for a sexually transmitted disease?
- Does your partner have HCV?
- Is your partner in a high-risk group for HCV?

HCV: Usually Incurable but Almost Always Controllable

The likelihood is that if you have had HCV in your system for more than six months, you will have it forever. Few people (only 20 percent) manage to expel the virus from their systems. Even aggressive long-term drug therapy is successful in less than half of all cases of chronic HCV.

Yet even in the majority of people who cannot overcome the chronic form of the virus, appropriate measures provide the opportunity to lead long, productive lives. In many cases, life expectancy is not affected at all. The key is your willingness to do what's necessary to keep the virus under control.

Once an accurate diagnosis is made, the most important goal is to begin an appropriate treatment program. These are the components of a successful program to manage HCV:

- Get the right medical treatment for your condition (chapter 3).
- Learn to live daily with your symptoms (chapter 4).
- Improve your spirituality (chapter 2).

The Psychological Impact of Hepatitis C

As with all chronic conditions, the psychological impact of HCV can be as devastating as the physical symptoms. The most common psychological symptoms are those associated with depression. They include the following:

- *profound, persistent episodes of sadness lasting for longer than two weeks*
- *loss of interest in favorite activities*
- *difficulty sleeping*
- *feeling depressed most of the day*
- *decreased sexual drive*
- *feelings of worthlessness*
- *difficulty concentrating*
- *absentmindedness*
- *recurrent thoughts of suicide*

Because these symptoms can be quite severe, HCV sufferers need health care beyond just medical treatment. Among the most common recommendations from doctors for people with these symptoms is to seek help from a mental health professional, such as a therapist, and to join a support group where members share common experiences and problems.

HCV: The Mind-Body Connection

Strong evidence suggests that spirituality is a fundamental component of extending survival rates for chronic illness. In addition to the physical benefits of prayer and meditation, which have been properly documented, practicing the principles of a spiritual program enhances a person's ability to cope emotionally with chronic conditions such as HCV.

Such coping skills are greatly needed. Because there are often no symptoms, or the symptoms are very mild, people who are diagnosed with HCV may have difficulty accepting either that they have the disease or that it has serious consequences for them. As a result, they may not take the necessary measures to address the disease. Learning to accept what we have no control over is an integral component of an effective spiritual program. If and when a person does accept he or she has HCV, emotions such as anger, frustration, anxiety, and depression are apt to surface. A spiritual program helps people get through these feelings.

The medical profession is beginning to recognize the need for a spiritual component in the management of chronic illnesses. Harvard Medical School is dedicated to studying the relationship between spirituality and illness. The doctors at the Mind/Body Medical Institute have discovered in laboratory studies that prayer and meditation actually benefit health. Although not all doctors are as open to including spirituality as part of the healing process, many in the health care profession are coming to acknowledge the great gift available to people with chronic illness who commit to exploring their spirituality.

Your Liver and Why It's So Important

Your liver is one of the largest organs in your body and one of the most important. It is located below your ribs on your right side and weighs about three pounds. Your liver is closely involved with many of your body's processes. That's why a disease such as HCV can have such a profound effect on your health.

These are some of the important functions your liver performs:

- *It detoxifies and neutralizes poisonous substances and chemicals in drugs, alcohol, pollutants, aerosol sprays, and so forth.*
- *It produces substances that help you resist infection.*
- *It filters out germs and bacteria from your blood.*
- *It controls cholesterol production and excretion.*
- *It produces bile to help your body absorb fat and fat-soluble vitamins.*
- *It helps controls blood clotting.*
- *It stores sugars, vitamins, and minerals.*

Cirrhosis and HCV

Cirrhosis is a condition in which healthy liver cells are damaged and become scar tissue. This process reduces the amount of healthy cells able to perform the various tasks the liver must do, especially breaking down food and drink so the body can absorb their contents. A damaged liver may cause widespread disruption of many bodily functions. The symptoms of cirrhosis include progressive fatigue, jaundice (yellow skin), icterus (yellow eyes), dark urine (the color of dark tea), abdominal swelling, muscle wasting, itching, disorientation and confusion, loss of appetite, and easy bruising.

Excessive alcohol consumption is the most common cause of cirrhosis. Drinking alcohol in excessive quantities puts an enormous strain on the liver, which can lead to damage and scarring of this important organ. Alcoholism may account for more than half of all cases of cirrhosis.

The next leading cause of cirrhosis is HCV. The damaging effects of the virus cause about one-third of all cirrhosis cases. If you have HCV, there is more than a 10 percent chance you will develop cirrhosis. Because of its potentially fatal effects, cirrhosis is one of the most undesirable consequences of contracting hepatitis C. If you have HCV, you can reduce the likelihood of developing cirrhosis through early detection, and, if accompanying tests reveal liver damage has begun, early drug treatment can help slow or stop further liver damage (drug treatment, however, is not used when cirrhosis is advanced).

Getting Help for Alcoholism

To help prevent cirrhosis from developing when you have HCV, it is also imperative that you abstain from alcohol. If you are or suspect you are an alcoholic and you have HCV, seek help to stop drinking. Inpatient and outpatient chemical dependency treatment centers exist nationwide. Ask your physician or therapist for a referral. Also, Alcoholics Anonymous has provided millions of alcoholics with the strength and hope they have needed to stay sober one day at a time. To find an AA meeting near you, look in the White Pages under "Alcoholics Anonymous."

CHAPTER TWO

A Spiritual Program to Help Manage Hepatitis C

Living with hepatitis C can be a challenge. Some of you may undergo lengthy bouts of drug therapy, which can be overwhelming. It can be all the more trying if the therapy doesn't work the first time around or during subsequent attempts. Just think: for a disease that may not be showing any symptoms, you could endure years of disruptive yet necessary drug therapy that has major side effects, including depression.

Developing the resolve you need to manage your HCV will require making some changes, not just to your daily routine but to the way you look at life. Making these changes can provide you with the opportunity to live a life that is more happy, joyous, and free—a life that may be better than you've ever known.

The question is, How do you go about this?

To achieve the resolve you need to successfully address your disease, you need a spiritual plan as well as a medical one. The Twelve Step program referred to throughout this book is such a spiritual program. It has worked with astonishing success for millions of people with the chronic illnesses of addiction, including alcoholism and drug addiction, gambling, and overeating. Its principles have provided great succor for people with other chronic illnesses as well.

The Twelve Step program is spiritual at its core. It is strictly nondenominational, however, and accommodates people of all faiths. The program also welcomes those who have no religious faith. Nevertheless, success in this program requires a profound change in thinking from self-centeredness to acceptance of a Higher Power beyond oneself.

How you see your Higher Power is a matter of personal choice. It does not have to be God in a traditional sense. If you asked individuals whose lives have been positively transformed by the Twelve Steps to identify their Higher Power, you would get a variety of answers. Many people would undoubtedly tell you that the most meaningful aspect of believing in a Higher Power is to be able to step outside themselves and to realize they are not the center of everything.

Twelve Step How-To

Thanks to the foresight of those who created the Twelve Step program, there is flexibility in this guide to better living with chronic illness. This set of principles makes no draconian demands on you but rather offers suggestions for behavioral changes that will result in an improved life with less emotional pain and greater spirituality.

There is no rule about how the Steps should be done. This is a matter of personal preference. Many people with chronic illnesses have experienced great improvement in their spiritual well-being by choosing to do the Steps selectively. The Twelve Steps build on each other, however. If you take the time to get a firm foothold on one Step before you go on to the next, you journey from acceptance to serenity one Step at a time.

Many people ask, Is there a time frame for doing the Steps? As long as it takes is probably the best advice. But it is important to feel you are making progress. As far as possible, you needn't feel stalled on one Step or take lengthy breaks between Steps.

And keep in mind that doing the Steps isn't a one-time thing. You continue to practice the principles of the Steps in your daily life, and there is nothing to stop you from starting again on Step One and working all the way to Step Twelve whenever you wish. For many people, "working the Steps" provides tremendous serenity and satisfaction, not to mention a simple plan for living well.

A careful reading of this part of this book will reveal

that the underlying concepts of the Twelve Steps are not unique. Those who developed the Twelve Steps simply reflected on how they got sober. But their experience is supported by the collective sagacity of philosophers, cultures, and religious leaders throughout the ages. You will soon see that the message in the Steps is ageless; the philosophy is timeless; and the strength and hope offered to those with chronic illnesses such as HCV is everlasting.

Much has been written about the Twelve Steps. The following pages will introduce you to each Step. If this is your first encounter with the Steps, you may find it helpful to gather more information. If you've been exposed to the Steps or currently work the program for an addiction, this chapter can serve as a review.

Step One: The Foundation of Recovery

We admitted we were powerless over chronic illness—that our lives had become unmanageable.

We've probably all heard it said that the first step is the hardest to take. This is certainly true with the Twelve Steps. In taking Step One, we must admit that we are powerless over HCV and that an important part of our lives—our health—is out of control. Who wants to do such a thing?

Step One gets us to face reality. We cannot alter the fact that right now we have a life-threatening virus in our bodies. This is something we must accept. We are powerless to change that fact.

If we have become consumed by the knowledge that we have a chronic disease—and are experiencing feelings of depression, anger, fear, and anxiety—then our lives have become unmanageable.

The First Step takes courage. We have to admit things about ourselves that we would prefer not to admit. Many of us have to see that our HCV is a consequence of choices we made in the past. Some of us have to accept that we contracted the disease through no fault of our own but that we now have to deal with the anger and other feelings we have as a result. Like thousands who have gone before us, we can summon the courage we need to take this Step, the first in our spiritual journey toward achieving the serenity we need to manage our disease in its entirety.

Step Two: A Promise of Hope

Came to believe that a Power greater than ourselves could restore us to sanity.

Spirituality is an integral part of any Twelve Step program for chronic illness. Why? Because finding the serenity and strength we need to manage this disease requires turning to a power beyond ourselves.

Many of us already believe in a Higher Power we call God. If we don't believe in a Power greater than ourselves, it's important we at least stay open-minded about the concept. Even the slightest amount of faith that a Higher Power can and will help us is better than no faith at all. If this proves difficult, we "act as if" we believe so we're open to experiencing its power.

Indeed, Step Two does not mean we must come to believe in God as presented in a formal religious context. If we think this is the case, we might dismiss the Twelve Step program because we think it won't work for us. Or, if we're religious, we may view the Steps as some sort of cult. We need to keep an open mind. Like all the Steps, Step Two is a suggestion from others who say, "This is the way it worked for us." These people have found that the Second Step gave them hope—and there is hope for us if we come to believe that the source of power we need lies outside ourselves.

If we were to ask everyone with HCV who has been restored to sanity how they identify their Higher Power, we would probably hear answers as varied as humankind's ideas on faith. Some might say God as they understand Him from the faith of their upbringing (the Christian God, for example); some may be more comfortable envisioning a female version of God; others might say God working through the Twelve Step program; and others might say their Power Greater was the Twelve Steps themselves, along with support group attendance and fellowship. A Higher Power is meaningful and personal, an entity with whom we find a powerful connection.

On Insanity

"Restore me to sanity? But I'm not insane!" That might be your response to the second part of Step Two. Insanity here refers to our tendency to steadfastly refuse to acknowledge our HCV—even after we've been told that unless we do something, we'll suffer deadly consequences. The *American Heritage Dictionary* defines "insane" as being foolish or absurd. Most people would agree that not taking the clear-cut measures necessary to control a life-threatening disease meets the definition of foolish or absurd.

Step Three: Turning It Over

Made a decision to turn our will and our lives over to the care of a Power greater than ourselves.

Of all the Steps, the Third Step can be the most effective in helping us transcend the emotional pain of chronic illness. Time and time again Step Three has provided what people have needed to get through difficult moments. It has helped them approach the management of their disease with remarkable resolve.

In Step One we admit we are powerless over the

fact that we have HCV, and we acknowledge that our disease has made our lives unmanageable. In Step Two we come to believe that a Higher Power can help us get through our emotional pain. Step Three is making the decision to let our Higher Power restore us from the emotional pain and unmanageability of our disease and to show us what we can do ourselves.

Turning our will over to a Power greater than ourselves doesn't absolve us from doing whatever is necessary to care for ourselves. Our Higher Power loves us whatever we do and helps us by showing us how to help ourselves. Our Higher Power speaks through others and through us. We learn to listen to our feelings and to act on them.

No longer will we try to force impossible solutions or beliefs that aren't in our best interest. We won't expend time and energy "willing" our disease to go away. We let our Higher Power determine the best way for us to handle our disease and all the emotions that go along with it.

It is the responsibility of each of us with HCV to cooperate with our Higher Power. We need to do all we can to improve ourselves physically, mentally, spiritually, and emotionally.

Turning our will and our lives over to the care of a Higher Power doesn't "cure" our HCV. But it does help us handle the challenge of managing our disease.

It gives us the ability to consider a plan or purpose higher than our own.

Achieving the balance between letting our Higher Power care for us and taking personal responsibility can be hard. We discover how to achieve this balance by communicating with our Higher Power through prayer and meditation. In this way the answers are often revealed.

Once we have begun the process of "turning it over," we begin to find the resolve to manage our HCV. We can halt, go inside ourselves, and in the tranquillity simply say the Serenity Prayer: "God, grant me the serenity to accept the things I cannot change, the courage to change the things I can, and the wisdom to know the difference. Thy will, not mine, be done."

Spirituality

Just what is spirituality, anyway? One thing it isn't is religion. Although many truly religious people are spiritual, and many spiritual people consider themselves to be religious, the two concepts are not one and the same. We don't have to be religious to be spiritual. Religion is a codification of society's relationship with God into rituals and institutions. Spirituality is our inherent relationship with ourselves, others, and a Higher Power.

Step Four: Knowing Yourself

Made a searching and fearless moral inventory of ourselves.

The importance of doing an inventory is to know ourselves better. By being searching and fearless about our liabilities, we gain insight into how we may have developed hepatitis C and why it is we react the way we do. Writing down our inventory helps us to understand what we need to do to correct the behaviors that brought us to this point and to understand which ways of living will best help us manage our disease.

In doing this Step, we must be moral but not moralistic. Our behavior has been good and bad—that is the reality. We must examine it. Make it ours. Many of us contracted HCV through no fault of our own, perhaps during a blood transfusion. But some of us developed the virus as a result of destructive behaviors such as intravenous drug use or unsafe sex with multiple partners. Neglecting our health was selfish and self-centered. Number one, we ignored the impact our poor health would have on our families. Think about it. We also need to examine our behavior since being diagnosed with HCV. We may have been refusing to acknowledge that our liver enzyme readings mean we're "really" sick—after all, we don't have any symptoms. And what about the impact emotionally? Have we indulged in excessive self-pity and ignored our doctor's recommendations? Have we taken our frustrations and displeasure out on our family and friends? Do we continue to drink alcohol?

In doing our inventories, we shouldn't restrict ourselves to aspects of our behavior having only to do with our HCV. It is important for us that we recognize flaws that may have nothing to do with whether we contracted the virus.

We mustn't punish ourselves for these behaviors. The goal is to know ourselves and to accept ourselves. Only when we see ourselves in a way that is enlightening, and not judgmental, can we strive to do better.

There are several ways to go about Step Four. The most common way is to use a straightforward, double-column list of specific positive and negative behaviors. Keep in mind that Step Four is not a test. We cannot fail it.

Taking the Fourth Step is a profound yet simple start to an ongoing way of daily living. It is the beginning of a path to self-awareness, a way to go today and each day hereafter. The inventory becomes a way of life based on the courage and willingness to be completely honest to oneself about oneself.

This self-assessment may be the most difficult feat of our lives. If we need encouragement, support, or help, we can ask for it from someone we trust, such as a chaplain or counselor, someone who will be nonjudgmental.

When we have completed our Fourth Step inventories, we will possess more self-awareness and self-acceptance. We're now ready for the Fifth Step. We're now ready to make some changes in our lives and in the ways we manage our disease.

Step Five: Telling My Story

Admitted to the God of our understanding, to ourselves, and to another human being the exact nature of our wrongs.

In the Fifth Step we openly, honestly, and willingly share who we are. This is a time for introspection as well as for laying ourselves bare. It allows us to let our Higher Power and another person see us for who we really are—flawed but lovable people capable of taking the measures necessary to manage our HCV.

Step Five gives us the chance to rid ourselves of the hidden side of ourselves, the side that sometimes causes us to feel shame.

We need to prepare for this Step. True self-awareness and honesty do not come easily to most people. We are used to avoiding our character defects. To stand and actually face ourselves as we truly are is a difficult and spiritually demanding proposition.

The key to a good Step Five is to have done a thorough, balanced, and honest Fourth Step. In particular, the rigorous self-honesty called for in Step Four helps us to gain the humility we need to do an effective Step Five.

To Admit to a Higher Power

With the help of a Higher Power, we can find the inner courage and strength we need to take the Fifth Step. Caring, loving, and forgiving, our Higher Power will help us realize that we are not the only ones who fall short.

To Admit to Ourselves

To admit to ourselves where we went wrong is a sign that we are practicing true self-honesty. But it isn't easy. Who wants to confess to character flaws that may have caused a chronic illness? We go through our lives ignoring the ways we inflicted damage on our own bodies. Really, though, we do not forget. The knowledge gnaws inside us.

Taking the Fifth Step without being totally self-honest is self-defeating. It merely perpetuates our negative feelings toward ourselves.

To do this Step well, it is important to love and to respect ourselves. Step Five allows us to reflect on whether we are coping with our disease in a loving and nonjudgmental way. It gives us the chance to accept ourselves as flawed human beings. It lets us understand that we need forgiveness and another chance at life.

When we forgive ourselves, we become free from the grip of guilt and shame.

To admit first to ourselves before admitting to another person shows we are willing to be really honest. We prove we are not afraid to face our real selves squarely. True honesty begins with this kind of self-honesty. Knowing ourselves and our strengths and weaknesses can profoundly help us overcome any perceived obstacles to managing our HCV.

To Admit to Another Person

We share the Fifth Step with another person. Why? Because sharing with another person the exact nature of our wrongs keeps us honest. By doing this Step, we allow another person to see us as complete, but flawed, human beings. Most of us will find this to be the hardest part of the Fifth Step. We may experience an overwhelming fear of embarrassment. But there is a great amount of relief in doing this. We no longer have to put energy into making others believe we're perfect.

Step Five is the opportunity to cast out those behaviors and traits that cause us emotional pain. It is not enough to acknowledge the nature of our wrongs to ourselves and through prayer to a Higher Power. It is only by speaking out, admitting out loud our mistakes, failures, and anxieties to another person that the feelings and deeds lose their power over us. For those of us with a chronic illness such as HCV, the Fifth Step is one major step away from a sense of isolation and loneliness. It is a step toward wholeness, happiness, and a real sense of gratitude.

Which "Human Being"?

During Step Five, most people wonder who they should share their secrets with. The fact is that almost anyone will do: a clergy person, a doctor, a psychologist, a family member who won't be adversely affected by our total honesty, a counselor, a friend, or even a stranger. The best candidates have the following qualities:

- *discretion*
- *maturity and wisdom*
- *willingness to share their own experiences*
- *familiarity with the challenges of a chronic illness*

Often such people are not readily available to us. One of our responsibilities in doing the Fifth Step is to look around carefully for someone who meets these criteria.

Whomever we decide to share our Fifth Step with, we must remember our intention is not to please that person but to heal ourselves. It is our inner selves that we are trying to satisfy.

We should also not be afraid of shocking listeners with our revelations.

Steps Four and Five Are Ongoing

The "housecleaning" process we do in Steps Four and Five is not meant to be a onetime event. As we will learn in Step Ten, regular personal inventories are measures we can take to help us transcend the emotional pain of our chronic disease and to better manage our condition. If and when we decide to do these Steps again, we do not need to go back over our whole lives unless we continue to carry anger or other unresolved feelings or realize we overlooked a behavior we would like to change. Otherwise, we pick up where we left off when we last took inventory. What is past is past. Whenever we take another Fourth and Fifth Step, it can become an opportunity for increased self-knowledge, self-acceptance, and learning to forgive and seek forgiveness as a way of daily living.

Step Six: Ready, Willing, and Able

Were entirely ready to have the God of our understanding remove all these defects of character.

In Step One we admitted we were powerless over whether we now have HCV. In Step Two we came to believe that our Higher Power could help us. In Step Three we made the decision to let that Power care for our lives. Steps Four and Five uncovered our defects of character.

If we have done these first five Steps honestly and thoroughly, we will be ready to let go of our character defects. The readiness to have them removed is the key to the Sixth Step. By being willing to let go of these character defects, we increase our chances of coping with our chronic illness.

In taking Step Six, we need to revisit that concept of powerlessness. Instead of telling our Higher Power what we want to be—"Make me more motivated" or, "Make me more open-minded"—we state our condition as it is. We state how things are with us: "My Higher Power, I am lazy" or, "My Higher Power, I am intolerant of others." Only with this humility will we be ready and willing to have such defects removed.

Even with all the preparation we do for the Sixth Step, we may still have reservations. Even when we know we no longer have any use for our defects of character, we've grown accustomed to them over the years. In our minds, our pride and selfishness served us well. We might ask ourselves, "Can I let go of some of my most monumental defects?"

That is why we go to the Seventh Step. It's there that we see our Higher Power doing for us what we really could not do for ourselves. For many, the removal of our shortcomings is the miracle that turns doubters into believers. Step Six is really the "get ready, get set" that builds toward the "go" of Step Seven—the action of asking our Higher Power to remove our shortcomings.

Step Seven: Being Changed

Humbly asked our Higher Power to remove our shortcomings.

The first word in Step Seven is "humbly." Because Step Seven so expressly concerns itself with humility, we need to stop to consider its importance.

Humility is the practice of being humble. It is the recognition of our self-worth and seeing that same God-given worth in other people, even when they are so totally unlike us that we don't understand them or get along with them. Humility is the awareness that we are not all-powerful controllers of every aspect of our lives and that we do need the help and guidance of a Higher Power.

"Humbly" asking our Higher Power is quite different from the way we may be used to praying—either begging or bargaining. In those cases we prayed to our Higher Power out of desperation. From now on we pray with humility; we humbly ask our Higher Power to remove our shortcomings.

Most people find it easier to ask that their shortcomings be removed gradually or one at a time. Having lived with these shortcomings for so long, we may find it difficult to shed them all at once. We need to be patient with ourselves and with our Higher Power during this process. This may take time and a lot of work on our part, before we are "entirely ready," as stated in Step Six. We don't expect to become perfect people, but we aim to improve. The goal is progress, not perfection.

We can work this Step alone with our Higher Power, with members of a religious group, or in support groups (for alcoholism, narcotics addiction, or HCV, for instance)—wherever we can trust and be trusted.

And although personal prayer may be our own connection with our Higher Power, when two or three are gathered together, we feel a special bond not only with our Higher Power but also with others who share our condition. We feel this closeness as we say the Serenity Prayer together in our groups.

Our own shortcomings can, with our Higher Power's help, be changed.

Step Eight: Preparing for Change

Made a list of all persons we had harmed, and became willing to make amends to them all.

Step Eight adds even more strength to our program. If we have harmed others, it is important to make a heartfelt attempt to reconcile with them and to release our guilt. If we have hurt friends and the friendships have suffered, the benefit is that we might repair those friendships. By making a list we become clear as to exactly whom we owe amends to.

Over the years some of our behaviors, such as drug use or drinking, may have caused discomfort to others—to family, friends, and co-workers. We may have been rude to them when they asked us to stop a particular behavior. Chances are that at the very least we ignored or rebuffed many people's feelings on the subject.

We might want to consider what our behavior was like after we found out we had HCV. It may have been unacceptable. We may have been disrespectful at times to the health professionals who were trying to help us with our recovery. Our list needs to include all persons we've harmed, regardless of how much and under what circumstances.

We may want to put ourselves at the top of our amends list. We are the ones whose health may be suffering as a result of our actions.

Understandably, the prospect of acknowledging our responsibility for hurting others can be daunting. As with the other Steps, Step Eight becomes less frightening once we settle down to do it.

We can take some time to write the names of a few people who make us feel uncomfortable. We don't need to write why or anything else. This simple act of writing down names changes our perspective. Instead of thinking about the harm others have done to us, we take responsibility for the pain we caused in those relationships. It is a profound experience that represents a coming of age.

If you made a list, congratulations. You are halfway through this important Step.

Many of us avoid the Eighth Step because we are already thinking ahead to Step Nine or because we feel too guilty or fearful to face a long list of names. It is important to remember that just because we've written a list does not mean we need to make amends immediately.

The second part of this Step involves willingness. Being willing to make amends means discarding all resentments and accepting responsibility for the harm we have done to others.

In so doing we become completely ready to do whatever we can to make amends for these harms, thereby unburdening ourselves of guilty feelings that interfere with our emotional well-being as we contend with our hepatitis C.

Continuing to Make Amends

The Twelve Step program is not a program of perfection. Instead, it stresses progress. Even when we practice the principles of this Twelve Step program in all our affairs, it is inevitable we will have "run-ins" with other people in our lives (though far fewer than before, it is hoped). For that reason a new and revised Step Eight list is an option for any of us at any time.

Step Nine: Facing the Past

Made direct amends to such people wherever possible, except when to do so would injure them or others.

We begin making amends to our loved ones by showing them we are caring for ourselves. In addition to protecting our livers against substances that might be harmful—and in general treating our bodies better— we follow our doctors' recommendations for drug therapy and submit to follow-up therapy when necessary. No longer do our families and friends have to fear we are, through inaction, killing ourselves. Many of our amends are made by the act of taking appropriate measures to contain our disease.

These, though, are "indirect" amends, and the operative word in Step Nine is "direct." Making amends directly helps us gain humility, honesty, and courage. That means we need to go directly to the people we have harmed and admit our wrongs. Being direct isn't just about righting wrongs. It also inspires us to summon honesty and courage to our service and gives us the freedom to look others in the eye and to experience the self-respect we deserve.

An amend need not consist of a lengthy explanation. All that's needed is a heartfelt apology. The person to whom we are making the amend may feel some uneasiness too. For this reason, simplicity and directness usually work best when making the amend.

Ideally we apologize face-to-face. The very directness of this approach is beneficial. Sometimes this is impractical, however, and we may choose to write a letter, make a phone call, or even, in this electronic age, write an e-mail.

In the vast majority of cases, amends are well received. Even in those rare instances when they are not, this is not a reason to avoid the effort the next time. Almost always, relationships improve markedly when amends are made.

Steps Eight and Nine also allow us to make amends to ourselves. The reward for taking these Steps is a gradual but increasing sense of self-acceptance and self-respect, of being in harmony with our own personal world. Such feelings are indispensable in our quest to cope better with the challenges of our chronic illness.

Step Ten: Maintaining Our New Lives

Continued to take personal inventory and when we were wrong promptly admitted it.

Managing our chronic illness presents us with a

tremendous challenge. Yet by following the Steps of this program, we have been able to achieve a strong measure of conciliation with ourselves, others, and a Higher Power. To help maintain our serenity, we must try to stay comfortable with ourselves and others. We do this by continuing to take a personal inventory.

We are only human. The path we are taking offers progress, not perfection, so it is inevitable—even with a Higher Power in our lives—that we will do things that we know are wrong or misguided. These can be monumental or trivial. Maybe if we have let our condition deteriorate to the point where distressing symptoms have begun, we entertained thoughts of suicide. Or the expense of a medication caused us to snap angrily at a pharmacist. When defects such as self-pity and anger rear up, we can go back and do a Seventh Step on them, asking our Higher Power to remove these shortcomings.

It helps to get feedback from people close to us—family, friends, fellow members of support groups. We need to ask these people to point out our character defects to us if they become apparent.

The second part of this Step emphasizes that if we want to maintain our serenity, we must admit our wrongs "promptly." It is important not to let anything build up inside us that will interfere with our program to cope with our chronic illness. Once we get used to it, admitting we're wrong can be a liberating sensation that enables us to move on in our lives without harboring resentments or other unhealthy thoughts.

Step Eleven: Partnership with a Higher Power

Sought through prayer and meditation to improve our conscious contact with a Power greater than ourselves, praying only for knowledge of our Higher Power's will and the courage to carry that out.

When coping with a chronic illness such as HCV, we need all the help we can get. The help of a Power greater than ourselves is available to us through prayer (talking to our Higher Power) and meditation (listening to our Higher Power). By praying and meditating in our daily lives, we keep a channel open to our Higher Power. We can rely on that Power's strength to help us at any time as we deal with the challenges of our disease.

Step Eleven calls for us to follow our Higher Power's will as it is revealed to us through prayer and meditation. Once we believe we are trying to do our Higher Power's will, we can ask for the strength to carry that out. When we do not feel like exercising or eating properly, we can ask for encouragement. When we have a compulsion to drink or smoke, we can ask our Higher Power to take it away. Our Higher Power is always with us and willing to come to our aid.

It's important for us to remember that although we

have turned over care of our disease to a Higher Power, we need to cooperate with that Power. By listening to others who share our condition, learning about our disease, and adhering to our doctors' advice, we are doing what is necessary to care for our hepatitis C and ourselves. And in so doing we will be better able to receive the strength that Power wants to provide.

The Importance of Prayer and Meditation

Medical science has demonstrated that prayer and meditation have a beneficial effect on our health (see page 19). These practices improve our health by helping us develop a closer relationship with our Higher Power, an improved "spirit consciousness."

Prayer is talking to our Higher Power. Meditation is listening to our Higher Power. Prayer and meditation don't come easily to everyone. As with most things, the more we do it, the better we get. Those who have cultivated a close relationship with their Higher Power can suggest ways that we, too, can pray and meditate. We need to seek out such people and consult them or read books on how to pray and meditate.

Perhaps the most oft-heard recommendation is to have a quiet time each morning during which we ask our Higher Power for the strength to manage our HCV that day and a similar interlude each night when we thank our Higher Power for helping us to live another day with our chronic illness.

Many people meditate for at least thirty minutes a day—a duration we may need to work up to. Meditation involves quieting the mind. We can begin meditating by getting in a comfortable position, closing our eyes, and focusing on a word, such as "peace." At first, many thoughts of what we "should" be doing enter our mind, but we learn to release them. When our minds are quiet, we are able to get in touch with our inner selves and to listen to our Higher Power. Afterward, sometimes miraculously, answers to our problems will just come to us.

The strength we need to cope with our chronic illness comes from communicating with our Higher Power in prayer and meditation. We must actively seek out spirit-communication with our Higher Power. This is a matter directly between us and that Power. From direct communication comes life, joy, peace, and spiritual healing.

Step Twelve: Carrying the Message

Having had a spiritual awakening as the result of these Steps, we tried to carry our message to others with our condition and to practice these principles in all our affairs.

By the time we reach Step Twelve, we've changed. The compulsion to deny our disease and to engage in behaviors that not only caused it but also made it worse has been lifted—not by our own power, but by a Power greater than ourselves. This in itself is a spiritual awakening that will help us as we contend with our disease.

If we've worked the Steps, we have the gift of being able to manage our chronic illness. If we haven't worked the program, we now know we have the tools.

Truly one of the best ways to keep this gift is to give it away. We have experience, strength, and hope that we can share with others. We let ourselves be used as a channel for a Higher Power to work through. We can now partake in the joy of helping others to live healthier, happier, and longer lives.

One way we might "give it away" is to make ourselves available as volunteers to those who organize HCV or drug prevention campaigns. Or we might provide comfort and company to people with HCV living in convalescent homes. If we attend Alcoholics Anonymous or Narcotics Anonymous meetings, we can help make the coffee, set up beforehand, and clean up afterward.

If we belong to an HCV support group and a member of our support group seems to be dwelling on the negative aspects of his or her life, we might spend some time with this person and try to lend a sympathetic ear and an encouraging word.

Whether or not we find an organized support group, we need to seek out and make friends with two or more people with HCV. We need to make it a point to have breakfast or lunch with them often, phone them regularly, and talk. We can praise their efforts and celebrate their successes (no matter how small) and let them do the same for us.

If we practice the principles of this Twelve Step program in all our affairs, we will likely realize our full physical potential with this disease and an abundance of spirit. We will live as our Higher Power intended us to—happy, joyous, and free.

On Spiritual Awakenings

For those unfamiliar with Twelve Step programs, the term "spiritual awakening" can be the subject of confusion. Many people assume that a spiritual awakening is by definition a cataclysmic occurrence—an opening of the heavens accompanied by a chorus of hallelujahs. In the absence of such an event, some of us might assume the program isn't working for us. But instant and dramatic conversions to spirit-consciousness are not what the Twelve Steps

are predicated on. Although such transforma-
tions take place, they are by no means the rule.
Most spiritual awakenings are simple, very
simple, yet the experience is profound. We feel
enlightened and in awe.

A spiritual awakening could be as simple as
a thought we have while walking through the
woods or watching a child. It could be suddenly
seeing ourselves or others in a totally different
light. It could be running into someone who
gives us the answer to the question we've been
asking ourselves.

A person may have one big spiritual awakening, but most people have many smaller-scale
awakenings. As the Twelve Steps become our
guide to living well with HCV and as we develop a relationship with a Power greater than
ourselves who loves us and cares for us, we
come to an understanding of what is truly meant
by the words "spiritual awakening."

To Alcoholics with HCV

If we are alcoholic, the challenge of coping
with HCV is especially difficult. Walking out
of the doctor's office after first being told we
have HCV, the first thing we might crave is a
drink. And our despondency in the wake of this
diagnosis might cause us to regularly seek out
alcohol. However, *if we have HCV and we con-*

sume alcohol, we face certain death from liver disease.

It may be constructive for alcoholics to think of it this way: being told we have HCV provides us with the immediate and irrefutable need to take the measures necessary to free ourselves from the grips of alcohol, something we probably wanted long before being diagnosed with HCV.

Step by Step

The advice in this chapter is primarily for those wishing to cope with the challenges of HCV itself. But the fact that it uses as its basis the Twelve Steps of Alcoholics Anonymous is a reminder to alcoholics that there is hope for us if we have the desire to stop drinking. Indeed, the Twelve Steps as used by men and women actively involved in AA support groups have proved to be one of the most effective ways to overcome the disease of alcoholism. If we are alcoholic, we can consider it crucial to seek help for our alcoholism. If we are active alcoholics with HCV—or recovering alcoholics who feel we might want to drink over the news that we have HCV—our need is all the greater. Help in the form of the Twelve Steps is available to us at local AA meetings. Reading this chapter will reinforce the lifesaving lessons you will learn in the fellowship of a Twelve Step program.

CHAPTER THREE

Medical Treatment for Hepatitis C

By practicing the principles of a Twelve Step program in your daily affairs, you will gain the resolve and serenity you need to treat your HCV and to live the rest of your life with the virus. Above all, you will learn to "turn over" your disease to the care of a Higher Power. You are now working with that Power.

Part of your responsibility to your Higher Power is to do all that is necessary to care for yourself and to adopt an assertive attitude toward your disease. If you have chronic HCV, it isn't going to just go away; you need to be proactive about keeping it at bay. Being proactive means finding an expert to treat you, starting and sticking with a vigorous drug regimen if necessary, coping with the sometimes debilitating side effects of that therapy, and accepting when a transplant is necessary.

Medical Care: Finding a Hepatitis Specialist

HCV is a complicated disease whose treatment is constantly changing. Your general practitioner cannot be

expected to be knowledgeable enough about or suffi-
ciently current on all aspects of caring for someone
with HCV, and he or she would probably be the first to
admit it.

If you have elevated liver enzymes and test positive
for HCV antibodies, your family doctor will refer you
to a physician who specializes in the treatment of
HCV—either a gastroenterologist or a hepatologist. (A
gastroenterologist specializes in diseases of the stomach, intenstines, and liver; a hepatologist specializes in
liver disease.) If your doctor does not provide you with
this referral, ask for one.

Once you understand your illness and have chosen a
particular therapy from among the options presented,
you should follow the treatment plan or discuss a change
in that plan with your doctor. You owe your doctors (and
yourself) honesty. If you stop taking your prescribed
drugs, consume alcohol, or start eating poorly, admit it.

Drug Treatment for HCV

It is crucial that you find out *as soon as possible* if you
need drug therapy. The timing of your treatment can
greatly affect its chances of success.

At present the most common drugs used to treat
chronic HCV are a combination of interferon and
ribavirin.[1] When used by itself, interferon works in 10

1. Ribavirin and interferon are generic names, as aspirin is a generic name for a type
of pain reliever.

to 20 percent of people. A combination of interferon and ribavirin works in about 30 to 40 percent of people. Ribavirin, when used alone, does not work against HCV. These drugs are used in a variety of combinations, depending on the person's specific condition. Other drugs are also being tested, and some of the results are promising. None of the drugs on the market are mood-altering and can therefore be considered "safe" for recovering addicts.

What is interferon and how does it work? When successful, this medicine slows the progression of the disease and damage to the liver by reducing the amount of virus in the body. (If you are diagnosed with "acute" hepatitis C, you'll most likely be treated with interferon immediately, as this can lower your risk of the disease becoming chronic and improve your chances of responding to the drug.) Interferon protects your healthy, uninfected cells from being invaded and taken over by the virus. In fact, interferon is an antiviral glycoprotein—a substance that is naturally produced by your body to help fight viruses. But sometimes your body may not produce enough interferon to fight virulent viruses such as HCV, in which case receiving additional interferon can help make the difference.

Who Should Be Treated with Drugs?

Anyone who develops chronic HCV may at some point need treatment with interferon or the combination of interferon and ribavirin. Because the side effects of such therapy can be severe, however, your doctor will probably prescribe drugs for you only if tests show you are developing liver damage. If you have chronic HCV but no signs of liver damage, the potential for unpleasant side effects may outweigh unknown benefits, and your doctor will probably hold off on prescribing drugs. In such cases, careful observation, including measuring liver enzymes regularly and getting a liver biopsy every three to five years, is an acceptable alternative to drug therapy.

The decision about drug therapy is less clear in other categories of people with HCV. You will probably be prescribed drugs for your HCV if blood tests and a liver biopsy reveal liver inflammation, aggressive HCV in your system, and the beginnings of liver damage.

If the virus has already seriously damaged your liver, you probably will not be prescribed drug treatment, as it will make you sicker without helping cure your disease. Drug therapy is not considered if you have cirrhosis.

Not enough studies have been done to determine whether to use drugs to treat HCV patients who are under the age of eighteen or over age sixty. If you have HCV and you belong to a patient group for whom there is no hard and fast rules on drug treatment, you need to carefully discuss drug treatment with your doctor. Ask your doctor to explain all the possible risks and benefits.

It is known that it's unsafe for the following groups of people to be prescribed interferon:

• women who are pregnant or who are planning to become pregnant soon
• patients with advanced cirrhosis
• patients with serious medical or psychiatric problems
• patients with fluid in the abdomen

Pregnancy and HCV

If you have HCV and become pregnant, tell your doctor immediately as it may affect the way you are treated. Keep in mind that if you want to get pregnant, interferon will interfere with your ability to conceive.

Pregnancy should not make your HCV worse. Your chief concern is that you will be healthy enough to carry your baby to term and get through the delivery. Fortunately, the risk of transmitting HCV from the mother to the unborn child is quite small (about 5 percent).

Your doctor will be able to tell you under what circumstances this could occur. In general, the baby will not contract the virus in the womb, but rather, during birth itself, and there is nothing that can be done to prevent this from happening.

If you are pregnant, *everyone* responsible for your health care needs to know that you have the virus, including the health care providers in the delivery room. This will help safeguard the health of your baby, the health of the people who'll be assisting in the delivery, and your health, since having HCV may mean you will need special care.

Most infants infected with HCV at the time of birth have no symptoms and are normal during childhood; however, more studies are needed to find out if these children will have problems caused by the infection. There are no licensed treatments or guidelines for treating infants or children infected with HCV. Children diagnosed with elevated ALT (liver enzyme) levels should be referred to a doctor who specializes in treating children with HCV.

There is no evidence that breastfeeding spreads HCV, though HCV-positive mothers may consider abstaining from breastfeeding if their nipples are cracked or bleeding.

Interferon Therapy: The Prescription

Interferon is usually administered by self-injection three times a week, and the treatment lasts for twelve months to two years. The two-year therapy has proved to lower early relapse rates, but it is expensive (more than $10,000) and the side effects are more severe. During drug therapy your doctor should carefully keep track of your liver enzyme levels (ALT) and antibody levels (HCV RNA) and do other tests to see if your liver is getting better.

The most recent research suggests that longer treatment is more likely to result in periods of remission and a lower risk of developing cirrhosis or liver cancer. This reinforces the need to continue taking the drugs your doctor has prescribed for as long as it takes to see if you are improving—even if the side effects are discouraging. After about three months, your doctor should be able to tell if the drug therapy is working. If it doesn't seem to be effective, you may be taken off the drug, or the doctor may change your dosage or alter your drug combination.

Follow-up is crucial. You must keep appointments with your doctor. When your course of treatment has finished, your doctor will again test for the presence of HCV and may measure its level using the HCV RNA blood test. Your doctor will also want to test you six months after the interferon therapy is complete. Even if tests cannot detect any signs of the virus in your blood, there is a 30 to 50 percent chance the infection will return from wherever it is lurking in your body. If this happens, you may need another course of treatment. In people who relapse, a second course of interferon treatment is often successful in reducing the virus so it never regains enough of a presence to cause symptoms. Second treatments usually continue for a long time—up to two years; however, your doctor may determine from the post-therapy tests that interferon will not work in your case. Sometimes, because of the genetic makeup of the virus you have, you may not respond well to drug treatment.

Side Effects of Drug Therapy

Most people who use interferon develop unpleasant side effects. Some, but not all, of these symptoms mimic the symptoms of HCV itself, which we learn to cope with in chapter 4. There are ways to lessen these effects, so you needn't use them as a reason to not participate in drug therapy. In any case, the side effects associated with drug therapy for HCV are usually the worst during the first few weeks of therapy and quickly become less severe. It is important, therefore, that if you are prescribed drugs to treat your HCV, you don't give up partway through your therapy. Your condition will improve! Call your doctor if you need help coping with these side effects. The Twelve Step program described in chapter 2 is an effective way to help you get through the difficult times associated with your medication.

Since the side effects of drug therapy are most severe during the first two weeks of the regimen, it's a good idea to take a week or two off from work if possible. Explain the situation to your boss if you think he or she will be sympathetic. If taking time off isn't practical, at least try to rest more. If you are responsible for keeping house and home, try to have others help with these duties. Consider paying for some temporary domestic help for the first week or two. People who have successfully completed an interferon program find that getting through the first two weeks is hardest. Get any necessary support during this time to greatly increase your chances of success in finishing the treatment.

The side effects of drug therapy for HCV are unpredictable. Not everyone who takes interferon gets side effects, and they occur in different combinations in different people. The most common side effects are flu-like symptoms: fatigue, fever, headache, muscle and joint aches, chills, and nausea. You may notice a metallic taste in your mouth and that food tastes different to you. Mild hair loss and itchy, dry skin are not uncommon. Interferon has also been linked to emotional and psychological changes such as irritability, apathy, and depression.

Coping with Drug Side Effects

Since interferon side effects are generally most severe four to six hours after the injection, consider injecting yourself just before bedtime. This will allow you to sleep through the worst of the side effects. Another suggestion is to adjust your injection schedule around your workweek. For instance, if you work Monday through Friday and you have been prescribed three injections a week, you can administer them Thursday, Friday, and Saturday. This way you will experience the worst of the side effects during only two of your workdays. Once you start a schedule, though, you must stick with it. If you follow the above recommendations, you may end up saying, "This isn't so bad after all."

The following are some additional ways to lessen side effects:

- Drink plenty of noncaffeinated fluids.
- Drink water and clear fruit juices immediately before and after your injection.
- Take over-the-counter pain relievers one hour before your injection (though some people have found taking one pill two to three hours *after* is even more effective).

Remember to always consult with your doctor before taking any over-the-counter or prescription medication for side effects. Combining alcohol and acetaminophen (an ingredient in many over-the-counter pain relievers and cold medicines) has been linked with potentially fatal liver failure, and people with HCV are especially at risk.

Also tell your doctor about all other medications you are taking for your health, including vitamins, supplements, and herbal remedies. Some of these may lessen the effectiveness of the interferon you are taking, while others may trigger harmful reactions. Your doctor should know about all other medicines you are taking while you are on interferon therapy.

- For headaches, try massage or a heating pad applied to the neck or simply lie down, close your eyes, and relax.
- It's extremely important to be well-nourished during drug treatment. For loss of appetite caused by nausea, try several small meals a day instead of three large ones; keep healthy snacks handy for when the urge to eat strikes. Much more on nutrition for people with HCV can be found in chapter 4.
- For fevers, try sponging yourself with lukewarm (not hot or cold) water.

- For a metallic taste in your mouth, try brushing your teeth several times a day or using mouthwash.
- For thinning hair, consult a hairdresser for tips on how to make your hair look fuller (those who work with an older clientele are usually more knowledgeable in this area). If the hair loss is more than you're comfortable with, consider experimenting with hats, caps, and scarves. When your drug therapy is complete, your hair will stop falling out and will grow back.

It's also important to be aware that interferon can cause psychological and emotional changes such as depression, irritability, and apathy. A spiritual program such as the Twelve Steps described in chapter 2 can help alleviate such conditions. Particularly important is participation in HCV support groups (for more on the benefits of support groups, refer to pages 78–79). Interferon has also been linked to cases of suicidal tendencies, which reinforces the need to be aware of the psychological effect the drug may be having on you.

You've been warned about the dangers of consuming alcohol if you have HCV. Ironically, the psychological changes that are sometimes brought about by interferon have been linked to relapses in alcohol consumption by recovering alcoholics (those who are abstaining from alcohol). The consequences of such a relapse if you are HCV-positive can be fatal. If you are a recovering alcoholic on interferon, you must be on guard against a relapse to alcohol. If you are participating in Alcoholics Anonymous, let your sponsor know your situation and tell your "home group" about it too. Both will help keep you sober. And never forget to make that phone call when you think you need help!

The same is true for recovering narcotics addicts—using interferon can trigger a relapse. Aside from the many troubles this will bring to your life, there is the added risk of yet another exposure to HCV through contaminated needles. Use the support of the Narcotics Anonymous program.

If you are an alcoholic or a drug addict and you are *not* a member of a Twelve Step program such as AA or NA, consider joining one. Twelve Step programs have helped keep millions of addicted people clean and sober.

What's Next?

Even if interferon doesn't improve your condition, you still need to work with your doctor to keep track of your disease. In particular, you need to know how much damage is taking place in your liver. If the damage becomes severe, you may need a transplant. Remember, though, that the time between infection and the need for a liver transplant can be as long as forty years. Even more important, keep in mind that if you take care of yourself, you may *never* need a transplant. The next chapter includes more information on coping with the symptoms of HCV and staying in good health. Liver transplants are described in chapter 6.

The Future of Treatment for HCV

The search for new treatments for HCV has been slow and often frustrating. But the need for more effective treatments is urgent, and many new approaches are being tried. Of the many treatment leads being pursued at this time, any one could be the next breakthrough.

Following are the most important areas of research.

Diagnosis

Better diagnostic tests will tell the doctor more about the particular kind of HCV infecting you, which will help with customizing your treatment. For example, certain strains of HCV are more susceptible to interferon than others.

Prevention

Improved prevention is another priority for researchers. Unfortunately, HCV is a difficult target for scientists trying to develop a vaccine. HCV can avoid detection and attack by a vaccine because the virus changes its genetic structure in a process called "mutation" (see page 12). In fact, HCV mutates so much that the body ends up having to fight several slightly different strains of the virus at the same time. This makes developing an effective vaccine very difficult.

An effective vaccine against HCV would have to protect simultaneously against many different strains of the virus. Developing different vaccines for each strain is unrealistic because there are far too many strains. Research on how to vaccinate against other diseases caused by mutating organisms—such as the flu or AIDS virus (HIV)—may help in developing a vaccine against HCV.

New Treatments

As discussed earlier, interferon and interferon in combination with ribavarin don't always work against HCV. The drugs work in less than half of all cases. Again, mutation seems to be the problem, as the disease is able to sidestep the treatment. One of the primary goals of scientists is to create a drug so powerful that it will overwhelm the virus no matter how much it mutates. Another problem is that the body produces antibodies against interferon when the drug begins to work, so scientists are trying to create forms of interferon that do not trigger antibodies.

Interferon works by strengthening the immune system and keeping the virus from infecting healthy cells. Other drugs being tested operate differently.

"Nucleoside analogs" are a group of antiviral drugs that insert themselves into the virus's genes and prevent it from reproducing.

"Protease inhibitors" are a family of drugs that interfere with the packing of viral genes into new viruses. Hepatitis researchers are encouraged by evidence that protease inhibitors designed to fight the AIDS virus have worked, which suggests that protease inhibitors may be effective against other mutating viruses such as HCV. But because protease inhibitors have to be custom designed to attack a particular virus, the class that works against the AIDS virus won't work against HCV.

On the positive side, the resources devoted to finding a cure for AIDS are paying dividends for people with HCV because many of the treatments for AIDS have applications for the treatment of HCV.

Combination Therapy

An area of research into HCV treatment that comes from AIDS research is "combination therapy." This form of therapy uses a mixture of different drugs all at once in the hope of preventing HIV from developing resistance to any one drug. Combination therapy has had some success in treating HIV. It has eliminated all measurable HIV from some AIDS patients' systems. Although it is not yet established whether the virus will return, this is the closest researchers have come to finding a cure for HIV.

Gene Therapy

Though doctors may have to wait several years before gene therapy is a reality, it is seen as the treatment of the future for HCV.

Gene therapy involves putting new DNA into a patient's tissues. The most encouraging form of gene therapy is known as "antisense therapy". This kind of gene therapy shuts off bad genes. The patient is given an artificial copy of DNA, an exact reproduction of a gene that the virus needs to reproduce itself. The antisense DNA attaches to the viral gene, interfering with the way it replicates and thereby killing it.

You can refer to the appendix (page 137) for many other sources of information about new treatments, including the American Liver Foundation and the U.S. Centers for Disease Control and Prevention.

Drug Abuse and HCV

If you're HCV-positive, you're cautioned against using alcohol, but it's also important to stay away from illegal drugs. If you use intravenous drugs, you can infect yourself with another virus, such as HIV, and you can infect others with HCV. Drugs also adversely affect or weaken your physical health, making your body less able to fight the virus. Furthermore, some studies have demonstrated that marijuana lessens the effectiveness of interferon.

Keys to Coping with Hepatitis C

- *Participate in a Twelve Step program of spirituality.*
- *Get the right medical treatment for your condition.*
- *Learn to live daily with your symptoms.*

CHAPTER FOUR

Daily Living with the Symptoms of HCV

It is common for people infected with HCV to have no symptoms. As a result, a large percentage of HCV-positive men and women are unaware they even have the virus. Still, many people with HCV *do* have symptoms. And in some people, the symptoms of chronic HCV become ongoing and severe, affecting nearly every aspect of daily life.

HCV symptoms may affect both people who have chronic HCV but who are not prescribed interferon because they don't yet have any liver damage and HCV-positive men and women who have unsuccessfully undergone interferon treatment.

Coping with the symptoms of HCV can seem overwhelming. That's why the first section of this chapter will address the emotional and psychological consequences of coping with a chronic illness such as HCV.

Emotional and Psychological Symptoms of HCV

Depression, anger, fear, and anxiety are among the most common emotional and psychological symptoms of having a chronic illness such as HCV. It's important to know how to recognize and cope with these symptoms.

Recognizing Depression

Learning you have HCV can hit hard. The knowledge that your life may never again be the same can cause feelings of loss and grief. It's common for people diagnosed with HCV to experience feelings of emptiness, hopelessness, and sadness. Then there is the loss of self-esteem, which may surface as feelings of uselessness, guilt, and shame. All these emotions are consistent with depression. Signs you have depression include a persistent feeling of sadness, not sleeping properly, loss of interest in activities you once enjoyed, and the inability to concentrate.

Depression may be short-term or could become severe, a condition known as "major depressive disorder." If symptoms persist for longer than two weeks or become noticeably more severe, tell your doctor. He or she may refer you to a mental health professional or prescribe antidepressant medication. Definitely speak to your doctor if you answer yes to four of the following questions:

- Do you feel sad, anxious, hopeless, or on the verge of tears for much of the day, every day?
- Have you lost interest in enjoyable activities such as eating, sex, and socializing?
- Are you eating more or less than usual? Have you gained or lost a significant amount of weight?
- Do you feel agitated, fidget constantly, or find yourself incapable of staying still?
- Are you always weary? Are you too fatigued to take on even small chores?
- Are you having problems concentrating?
- Have you had thoughts of wanting to die?

Interferon can cause depression, but this is temporary and usually affects you only during your first few weeks on the drug. Antidepressants are usually not prescribed in such cases because the depression is probably not going to be permanent. However, chemical changes in your body may cause depression. This condition may require antidepressants to alleviate it. The doctor treating your HCV needs to know about any antidepressants you are taking.

Recognizing Anger

It doesn't matter how you became infected with HCV; chances are that when you find out you have the disease, you will be angry. If you got it through a transfusion, you may be angry at the hospital where you had the procedure. If you got it through intravenous drug use, you will be angry at yourself or other drug addicts around you at the time. If you got it through sexual contact, you could be angry at the person who gave it to you or angry at yourself for not taking the necessary precautions.

Recognizing Fear and Anxiety

Fear is an inevitable part of having a chronic illness, and HCV is no exception. There is the fear of the unknown—not knowing how your disease will progress and whether drug treatment will work; the fear of rejection by friends and family; and the fear that having a chronic illness could affect your employment or your finances. Anxiety resembles fear. Anxiety includes feelings of nervousness or tension in response to a particular situation—in this case, having the chronic illness HCV.

Following are symptoms associated with anxiety:

- Mental: impatience, restlessness, tension, problems concentrating, difficulty sleeping, and loss of enjoyment of pleasurable activities
- Physical: dry mouth, nausea, sweating, dizziness, diarrhea, constipation, muscle aches, sexual difficulties, rapid heartbeat, and shortness of breath

Coping with Emotional and Psychological Symptoms

Negative feelings can serve a purpose. They can get us to take on a new perspective, to see life from a different point of view. But if we dwell on our negative feelings for too long, they can cause needless suffering. There are several ways to overcome negative feelings.

Finding Help

Participating in a Twelve Step program is one way to help deal with intense feelings. (A Twelve Step program to cope with HCV is described in chapter 2.) Working the Steps has helped millions of people overcome feelings of depression, anger, fear, and anxiety associated with chronic illness.

It may also be necessary to seek help from a mental health professional, especially if negative emotions start to overwhelm you. If you've never been to a therapist, you may be reluctant at first. You may think you're strong enough to handle it on your own. You may fear that others will see you as weak. It's helpful to know that the stigma once associated with seeing a therapist is fading, and the results of seeking professional help can be profoundly beneficial if you're suffering emotionally. A therapist who counsels those with chronic illness—preferably people with HCV—can help you find ways to cope with the emotional and psychological challenges of your disease. A therapist will help you discuss your concerns about your disease, show you how to get involved in enjoyable activities, and suggest ways to channel your energies positively.

A therapist can also direct you to an HCV support group. Finding a support group is important for anyone who has HCV. Even when you know that you are one of millions of people with HCV, sometimes there's a tendency to feel you're going through this alone.

What Is a Support Group?

Support groups consist of people who have come together to share the common experiences and problems unique to their disease or condition. In addition to being a place to meet people who share a common bond, self-help and support groups also help members in other ways. Through newsletters and regular contact with other people in similar situations, members receive up-to-date information regarding their disability and treatments that are available. Along with this sharing comes understanding and a sense of belonging. Research confirms that the coming together of people in trouble serves to increase self-esteem, decrease anxiety and depression, and raise levels of overall well-being.

Information on support groups in your area

can be found in a variety of ways. Local news-
papers often offer feature listings. Handbooks of
community resources that sometimes include
support groups are usually available in local libraries and hospitals. Particularly active groups
are often listed in the Yellow Pages under "social
service agencies." Major national groups such as
the American Liver Foundation can provide you
with information about support groups in your
area and tell you how to start one of your own.

As soon as you begin your drug regimen—or even if
your doctor decides your condition is not yet severe
enough that you need such therapy—you should seek
out an HCV support group, even if you don't believe
support groups are for you. The relief that comes from
sharing thoughts, feelings, and coping strategies with
people who are in the same position as yourself can be
monumental. Don't discount the importance of these
groups before you've given them a fair chance. Attend
at least six meetings with an open mind before you decide whether they're for you.

A support group usually meets at least once or
twice a month for one or two hours at a time. Although
some people recommend that a therapist be present to
guide the discussion, many groups (including Twelve
Step programs such as Narcotics Anonymous) offer

excellent support for their members without paid professionals present.

The role of a therapist in an HCV support group is in part to make sure that the discussion does not focus on the negative. In a group without a therapist present, participants must remember that while a support group is a place to share hardships, the emphasis is on the positive progress participants have made since starting therapy. Certain meetings should be set aside for spouses and family members to attend also.

Maybe there are no support groups in your area, in which case think about starting one yourself. Get advice about starting a support group from a group therapist at your local community services organization.

You may decide to use the Twelve Steps as the basis for the support group you form. Why not? After all, the Steps have been used with extraordinary success by people dealing with a variety of other chronic illnesses. If you decide to make yours a Twelve Step group, learn how to run it by talking to the Alcoholics Anonymous World Services office in New York or from someone who is very familiar with Twelve Step groups. A longtime member of Alcoholics Anonymous, Nicotine Anonymous, Overeaters Anonymous, or Al-Anon (a Twelve Step program for family members and adult children of alcoholics) would be ideal. That person might recommend you also incorporate the Twelve

Traditions of AA as guidelines for how to organize your group. You may also want to consider getting involved in one of the many Internet "chat rooms" available for people with HCV.

Through a support group, and by communicating and interacting with others who share your disease, you may discover that having HCV has presented you with the opportunity to address issues which would otherwise have remained unmanaged and which, having been dealt with, will make you a more complete person.

Getting Informed

A fear of the unknown is behind many of the negative feelings associated with chronic illness. So it's important to learn as much as you can about your disease. Reading this book is a good start. There are other excellent published sources of information about HCV, but be sure to seek out those that address the emotional and psychological issues of having a long-term disease.

If you haven't done so already, find physicians who are knowledgeable about HCV, such as gastroenterologists or hepatologists, and find out from them about treatment options.

Another useful source of information is the Internet. If you have a telephone line and a computer, then the vast resources of the Internet are available to you in the comfort of your home. Otherwise, many libraries have computers that are hooked up to the Internet for use by library members. Once you are online, access to most medical research resources on the Internet is free. Some sites take the latest medical research and "translate" it into lay terms. Lessons in the basics of using the Internet are widely available. Classes may be held at your local library, senior center, or adult learning center. Keep in mind that many sites on the Internet offer dubious information, so be a discriminating net surfer. Refer to the appendix (page 137) for a list of legitimate organizations that have Internet sites.

Learning Stress-Management Techniques

Learning you have HCV and living daily with the disease can be extremely stressful. Not only is being stressed out unpleasant; it is also unhealthy and may worsen your medical condition. You will benefit by learning skills to decrease the stress in your life and, whenever possible, by removing yourself from situations currently stressful to you.

Following are some simple ways to deal with stress:

- Exercise. (See pages 85–89 for a beginner's walking program.)
- Take time to relax with a good book, movie, or music.
- Develop new interests, or rekindle your interests in past activities (take a course).

- Interact—spend time with family and friends.
- Address a person or situation that's causing you to react stressfully.
- Join a support group.
- Learn about your disease, but don't obsess about it.

One of the most effective ways to deal with stress is prayer. Praying evokes the "relaxation response"; it decreases blood pressure, heart rate, and breathing rate. A short invocation known as the Serenity Prayer can be said anytime you feel stress:

> God, grant me the serenity
> To accept the things I cannot change,
> The courage to change the things I can,
> And the wisdom to know the difference.

Prayer is not the only way to evoke the relaxation response. Some of the dozens of other relaxation techniques—such as meditation—are centuries old. Others, such as progressive relaxation and biofeedback, have been developed only in the last few decades. If living with HCV is causing you extreme stress, then the more methods of relaxation you know, the better. Compare relaxation to fitness: the more forms of exercise you can do, the easier it is to stay in shape. Different exercise modes can be employed in different situations and moods. The same goes for relaxation.

The National Institutes of Health recognizes a variety

of methods to reduce stress, including prayer, support group attendance, yoga, and biofeedback. Among the most common relaxation techniques are "deep breathing" and "meditation."

Deep Breathing

Deep breathing is one of the simplest and most effective ways to relax. It is also one of the most practical methods of relaxation because you can do it almost anywhere. Deep breathing is also a component of many other relaxation and meditation techniques, making it a good skill to master. Here is one breathing technique you can use:

- Sit up straight or lie flat on your back.
- Breathe in slowly through your nose and imagine you are pushing that air deep into your belly.
- Note how your belly expands as your lungs fill with air.
- Now breathe out slowly through your mouth.
- Continue breathing in this way, watching how your belly rises and falls.
- Do this twice a day for five minutes at a time.

Meditation

Like deep breathing, meditation can be done almost anywhere, although most people prefer, and beginners may need, peace, quiet, and solitude. Meditation has been described as intense and inward-focused concentration that allows you to focus on your senses, step back from your thoughts and feelings, and perceive each moment as a unique event. Meditation puts you in a rest state. You actually rest more deeply when meditating than when sleeping. Generally, meditation can be classified as two different types: "concentrative" and "mindfulness meditation."

In concentrative meditation you use a picture, word, or phrase (mantra), object (such as a candle flame), or a sensation (such as breathing) to focus the mind. If your mind begins to wander, you refocus your attention on the item you have chosen.

Mindfulness meditation is more complicated. Instead of focusing on a single sensation or object, you allow thoughts, feelings, and images to float through your mind. You let these thoughts go in and out of your mind without expressing positive or negative feelings about them.

Find out more about meditation and other relaxation techniques by reading books on the subject or by taking classes. Discover which relaxation techniques work best for you, and make them part of your day.

A Beginner's Walking Program

Exercise is a simple way to deal with the stresses of living with a chronic illness. The beginner's walking program is designed for people who haven't exercised for some time. Even if you are very unfit, you can do the walking sessions described in the early part of the program. Each walk session is divided into three parts: the warm-up phase, the target zone phase, and the cool-down phase. Of these three phases, the target zone requires explanation.

Achieving the Target Zone

To get the maximum benefit from exercise, it is necessary to exercise hard enough that your heart and lungs are working at between 60 and 75 percent of their maximum capabilities.

To see if your heart rate is within your target zone, you need to check your pulse while you're exercising. Here's how:

- *Place the tips of your fingers over one of the major blood vessels (try just to the left or right of your Adam's apple or the spot on the inside of your wrist below the bone of your thumb).*
- *Count the number of times your heart beats during a ten-second period. Then multiply that number by six to figure out how many times a minute your heart is beating.*
- *Compare your heart rate with the chart on the following page. For instance, if you are sixty-five years old, your goal is to have a target zone of between 78 and 116 beats per minute.*

Age	Target Heart Rate Zone
20 years	100–150 beats per minute
25 years	98–146 beats per minute
30 years	95–142 beats per minute
35 years	93–138 beats per minute
40 years	90–135 beats per minute
45 years	88–131 beats per minute
50 years	85–127 beats per minute
55 years	83–123 beats per minute
60 years	80–120 beats per minute
65 years	78–116 beats per minute
70 years	75–113 beats per minute

	Warm-Up Phase	Target Zone Phase	Cool-Down Phase	Total
Week 1				
Session A	Walk normally, 5 min.	Walk fast, 5 min.	Walk normally, 5 min.	15 min.
Session B	repeat	repeat	repeat	repeat
Session C	repeat	repeat	repeat	repeat

Each week do the walking session three times, as shown for week one. If you find you reach a point where the sessions leave you overly fatigued (tired enough that you don't think you could go to the next level), repeat that week's program until you think you are fit enough to move on to the next level. You don't have to complete the program in twelve weeks.

	Warm-Up Phase	Target Zone Phase	Cool-Down Phase	Total
Week 2	Walk normally, 5 min.	Walk fast, 7 min.	Walk normally, 5 min.	17 min.
Week 3	Walk normally, 5 min.	Walk fast, 9 min.	Walk normally, 5 min.	19 min.
Week 4	Walk normally, 5 min.	Walk fast, 11 min.	Walk normally, 5 min.	21 min.
Week 5	Walk normally, 5 min.	Walk fast, 13 min.	Walk normally, 5 min.	23 min.
Week 6	Walk normally, 5 min.	Walk fast, 15 min.	Walk normally, 5 min.	25 min.
Week 7	Walk normally, 5 min.	Walk fast, 18 min.	Walk normally, 5 min.	28 min.

	Warm-Up Phase	Target Zone Phase	Cool-Down Phase	Total
Week 8	Walk normally, 5 min.	Walk fast, 20 min.	Walk normally, 5 min.	30 min.
Week 9	Walk normally, 5 min.	Walk fast, 23 min.	Walk normally, 5 min.	33 min.
Week 10	Walk normally, 5 min.	Walk fast, 26 min.	Walk normally, 5 min.	36 min.
Week 11	Walk normally, 5 min.	Walk fast, 28 min.	Walk normally, 5 min.	38 min.
Week 12	Walk normally, 5 min.	Walk fast, 30 min.	Walk normally, 5 min.	40 min.

Week 13 onward: Remember to check your pulse periodically during the target zone phase to make sure you are exercising in that zone. As your lungs adapt to the demands of this walking program, try exercising in the upper range of your target zone. Gradually increase your fast-walking time to between thirty and sixty minutes three or four times a week. With a five-minute warm-up and cool-down period, your walking sessions should last forty to seventy minutes.

Physical Symptoms of HCV

Many people with HCV have no symptoms for many years after first being infected, but a lot of people *do* suffer symptoms early on. Attending to the emotional and psychological consequences of your HCV—as described in the previous section—is important because it will help with the physical symptoms. It's also necessary to deal directly with the symptoms themselves. You may experience varying degrees of HCV symptoms, and in different combinations from other HCV-positive men and women. If your HCV is successfully treated with drugs, your symptoms will go away.

The following section contains information about the most common symptoms of HCV infection and ways to cope with them.

Fatigue

By far the most common symptom of HCV is fatigue. There are ways you can lessen feelings of tiredness. One of the most effective of these, paradoxically, is exercise. Staying fit will give you endurance to counteract the fatigue.

If you have HCV, there is no form of exercise you are not supposed to do. You can play tennis, do aerobics, swim, and lift weights. The level of intensity depends on certain factors. Most important is your level of fitness. If you are in shape, there's no reason to cut back on your exercise regimen because you have HCV. If you haven't exercised for a long time or you are unfit, however, you need to start slowly. A walking program may be ideal for you if you think you need to start slow.

It's also important to develop and stick to a schedule. In addition to making exercise a part of your life, you also need to get enough rest. An afternoon nap may help give you the boost you need, provided it does not cause you to stay up at night. If you're having trouble getting a full night's sleep every night, let your doctor know. Lack of sleep is often associated with stress, so try to lessen the stress in your life, and certainly try to make sure you don't go to bed tense and anxious. Learn stress management techniques to help you with this (see pages 82–85).

Headaches

HCV and its drug treatment can cause headaches. These headaches may come and go and may vary in severity. Fortunately, headaches associated with HCV are easily treated with over-the-counter pain relievers. Again, check with your doctor before you use any such medication. Other causes of headaches are dehydration and tension; make sure you drink enough fluids (see pages 106–7) and if necessary practice stress management techniques (see pages 82–85) if you think stress may be contributing to your headaches.

Nausea and Loss of Appetite

It's not uncommon for HCV-positive people to complain about nausea. Usually this is accompanied by loss of appetite. Good nutrition is very important if you have HCV. This is described in greater detail in chapter 5. Some tactics to help counter loss of appetite that have been used successfully by people with HCV are as follows:

- Eat several smaller meals during the course of the day instead of three large ones.
- Eat a larger meal in the morning, as nausea is usually less severe earlier in the day.
- Certain foods are easier to stomach than others. Try eating foods you would eat when recovering from the flu, including dry crackers, broth, Jello, mashed potatoes, or plain pasta.

If your nausea becomes severe, or if you are throwing up, tell your doctor. Medication may be available to stimulate your appetite.

Joint and Muscle Aches

Aches and pains in the joints and muscles are frequently experienced by people with HCV. Over-the-counter pain relievers can help with the discomfort, which in many cases mimics arthritis. Remember, though, to speak with your doctor before taking any medication, as it may put a strain on your liver. If you suffer from muscle and joint aches and pains, ask your doctor what types of pain relievers will help you, how much you can take, and for how long. If you are an addict or alcoholic, ask your physician or pharmacist to be sure you're not taking medication that could be addictive.

About one-third of HCV-positive men and women experience "cryoglobulinemia"—joint and muscle pain caused by antibodies that develop in response to hepatitis C. If you have joint or muscle pain, tell your doctor and he or she may want to test you for cryo-globulinemia, which can cause problems in the circulatory system.

There are many strategies you can use to relieve the emotional, physical, and psychological symptoms of your HCV. Using the Twelve Step spiritual program described in detail in chapter 2 can help keep you in the right frame of mind.

A Twelve Step spiritual program shows you that you have to accept you are HCV-positive before you can deal with your disease effectively. You turn over care of your disease to a Higher Power and dedicate yourself to cooperating with that Power. By following a Twelve Step program, you learn to work for your Higher Power, with your Higher Power, and through your Higher Power. "Working the Steps" has helped millions of people with chronic illnesses to effectively manage their disease.

Refer to the Twelve Steps of Alcoholics Anonymous, adapted for use by persons with the chronic illness of HCV, on pages xxi–xxii.

Telling Others You Have HCV

So many misconceptions exist about HCV, and there is still a stigma attached to having the disease. Many people believe it's caused by drug addiction and that it's contagious. It can be a daunting prospect revealing that you have HCV, especially to close friends and family. Many people find they are ashamed to admit they have this disease.

It is important that you tell those close to you, however. Their support and understanding will help you cope with the physical, emotional, and mental challenges of this chronic illness. Also, you will need their help when you are not up to performing certain tasks such as housework or running errands and when you need help getting to the doctor's office, avoiding alcohol, eating healthily, and making sure you have the right medications on hand. Of course, you need to tell others so they won't inadvertently catch the virus from you.

Whom should you tell you have HCV? Three recommendations are

- people you trust
- people who care about you
- people who are in the position to help you

People tend to be afraid of what they don't understand, so when you tell others you have HCV, it is important to provide them with solid, accurate information. Letting them read this book may be a help. In the meantime, it's important you cover three important topics with your confidants:

- what the symptoms may be and how you might be affected
- what, if any, treatment you will be having and what the side effects of the treatment may be
- what the risk is of infecting others with HCV[1]

HCV in the Workplace

If telling a friend or family member is difficult, then informing people at work that you have HCV may seem out of the question. Yet this is something that deserves careful consideration, as you probably can and need to keep your job as you manage your disease.

In general, use the same criteria for telling your colleagues as your family: tell those whom you trust, those who care about you, and those who can help you.

1. Remember to stress that the risk of transmission is very low because the virus can only be transmitted through blood and cannot be transmitted through casual contact such as hugging, holding hands, or kissing.

What about your employer? This is a difficult question. Before you make your decision, consider how having HCV might affect your job. Ask your doctor whether you are putting others at risk in your place of work. The risks of transmitting the disease to others in the workplace is small.

There are pros and cons to telling your boss. On the plus side, he or she will understand your situation better and may be able to help you cope and continue in your employment. But there may be a downside if your employer adopts a negative attitude. Fortunately, there are federal and state laws that protect you. The federal Americans with Disabilities Act (ADA) protects you from being fired or pressured to quit because of your condition—as long as you can continue doing your job despite your illness. This doesn't mean you won't be fired or discriminated against if you tell people at work about your condition; it simply means you have a right to sue if your employer does not obey this law.

The ADA: A Primer[2]

Your employer cannot legally discriminate against you because you have HCV. According to the Americans with Disabilities Act, employers cannot legally

---

2. Employers with fewer than fifteen employees are not bound by the ADA.

- *limit your opportunities or status*
- *institute company policies that discriminate against you because you have HCV*
- *refuse to make reasonable changes to help you continue to do your job*
- *use your disease as an excuse to prevent you from doing some aspect of your job*

In addition, a prospective employer cannot ask you questions about your condition during the job interview.

To claim your rights under the ADA you must be able to perform the essential functions of your job, and you must have told your employer about your condition.

If you believe your employer is violating the law, you can contact the local branch of the Equal Employment Opportunity Commission (EEOC), which handles ADA complaints. You can also contact the Department of Justice, which operates the ADA Mediation Program, to try to resolve such problems. If you can't reach a resolution, you can still sue under the provisions of the ADA.

If you decide to reveal your condition to your employer, you need to decide whom to inform. You may want to start with the human resources or medical department, if your company has one. If you decide to tell your boss, choose a calm time at work to ask for a private moment. Try to anticipate any questions he or she might have and consider bringing along this book or an informational brochure. In particular, be ready to answer questions from your boss about how the disease might affect your job performance and what the likelihood is of transmitting the disease to your co-workers.

For specific advice on your situation, you should consult a lawyer in your area. The local American Bar Association may be able to help you find one who specializes in disability law.

Using the Family Leave Act

The Family Medical Leave Act (FMLA) provides that if you have worked full time for a company for a year or more, you can take up to twelve weeks of unpaid leave every year to attend to serious medical problems. The time can be taken all at once or in increments. Your spouse or another family member can also take this time if your condition is serious enough that he or she needs to care for you. Make sure you speak with your boss about the FMLA before you take any time off. In addition to the federal FMLA, many states have laws that provide similar protection.

How Can I Prevent Spreading HCV to Others?

- *Do not donate your blood, organs, other tissue, or sperm.*
- *Do not share personal-care articles that may have your blood on them, such as toothbrushes, dental picks, and razors.*
- *Cover any cuts or open sores on your body.*
- *If you have one long-term, regular sex partner, the chances of giving HCV to that person are slim. In such cases you probably don't need to change your sexual practices. The Centers for Disease Control doesn't advise changing sexual habits or using condoms in long-term monogamous relationships. A partner who doesn't have HCV by the time the infection is diagnosed probably won't get it. If you have multiple sex partners, you should always use latex condoms during sex.*

HCV is *not* spread by

- *breastfeeding (unless nipples are cracked or bleeding)*
- *sneezing*
- *hugging*
- *coughing*
- *sharing eating utensils or drinking glasses*
- *food or water*
- *casual contact*

CHAPTER FIVE

The Importance of Good Nutrition

If you have HCV, it's important that you stay as healthy as possible to fight the infection and its side effects. Eating well is one of the most effective ways to build your body's defenses. Having HCV, however, can actually interfere with your ability to practice good nutrition. Side effects may cause you to lose your appetite, and food may actually seem offensive to you. The depression that often accompanies a chronic illness may also affect your appetite. It may cause you to turn to alcohol to cope with your anguish.

What you put into your body will dramatically affect how your body responds to HCV. This chapter will provide you with nutrition recommendations to help you cope better with your HCV.

The Basics of Healthy Eating

Healthy eating means a balanced diet containing a variety of foods that provide you with all the important nutrients your body needs every day to work properly.

Good nutrition is a fundamental component of treatment for men and women with HCV who do not already practice healthy eating.

If your appetite hasn't been affected by HCV, then you can follow established guidelines for good nutrition. The food guide pyramid provided by the U.S. Department of Agriculture (USDA) is an excellent guide to eating a balanced diet. It is a simplified, systematic way to ensure an adequate intake of calories and all essential nutrients that avoids the need to calculate exact amounts of protein, minerals, and other substances that are needed every day. It goes beyond the "basic food groups" once promoted by nutritionists and other health professionals. The food guide pyramid is based on the USDA's research on what foods Americans eat, what nutrients are in those foods, and how individuals can make the right food choices. The pyramid helps people choose what and how much to eat from each food group to help keep fat intake and saturated fat intake low. A diet low in fat reduces the chances of getting certain diseases and helps maintain a healthy weight. The pyramid helps individuals learn how to spot and control the sugars and salt in their diets and helps people choose foods with less sugar and salt.

For a resource that describes the food guide pyramid in detail and shows you practical ways to eat healthily, log on to the USDA's Web site at www.usda.gov and read about the food guide pyramid online.

Meanwhile, here are the basics of using the food guide pyramid.

What to Eat: The Food Guide Pyramid in Brief

Bread, cereal, rice, and pasta: Choose six to eleven servings of bread, cereal, rice, and other grains daily. Include some whole grains, such as whole wheat or enriched bread or bran cereal. Any one of the following is equivalent to one serving of grain:

- 1 slice of bread
- 1 ounce of read-to-eat cereal
- $1/2$ cup of cooked cereal, rice, or pasta

Fruit: Choose two or more servings of fruits (including fruit juices) daily, including one good source of vitamin C, such as orange juice. Any one of the following is equivalent to one serving of fruit:

- a medium banana, apple, or orange
- $1/2$ cup cooked, canned, or cut-up fruit
- $3/4$ cup of juice

Vegetables: Choose three or more servings of vegetables daily, including at least one serving of a dark, leafy green or dark orange vegetable, such as

- ½ cup cooked carrots or chopped vegetables
- 1 cup of raw leafy vegetables, such as lettuce or spinach
- ¾ cup of vegetable juice

Meat, poultry, fish, dry beans, eggs, and nuts: Choose two to three servings equaling five to seven ounces daily of meat, poultry, fish, and other protein foods, such as beans, eggs, tofu, and unsalted nuts. Any of the following is equivalent to one serving of meat, fish, or poultry:

- 2 to 3 ounces of cooked lean meat, poultry, or fish
- 1 egg
- ½ cup tofu
- ½ cup cooked beans
- 2 tablespoons peanut butter

Milk, yogurt, and cheese: Choose two to three servings of milk, cheese, or yogurt daily. Any one of the following is equivalent to one serving of a dairy product:

- 1 cup milk
- 1 cup yogurt
- 1½ ounces of cheese

Salt: A Special Danger

Because salt increases fluid retention, avoiding salt is especially important if you experience fluid-related swelling associated with your HCV.[1] Most Americans eat much more salt than they need. Current recommendations are to consume no more than six grams a day of sodium—about one teaspoon of table salt. If HCV causes you to have fluid retention, you should probably try to consume even less sodium.

Few people add this 2,400 milligrams of salt to their food at the table each day, yet they are getting it in their diet. How? Most of the salt we eat is a natural part of the food itself, or more often, it's mixed in during its preparation, usually in fast foods or processed items.

Here are some tips to make sure you do not consume excessive sodium:

- One easy way to cut back on salt is simply to remove the saltshaker from your table.
- Check food labels for sodium contents. Favor foods lower in sodium. Look for packaging that indicates the contents are lower in sodium ("sodium-free," "very low sodium"). Buy low- or reduced-sodium or "no-salt-added" versions of foods that are typically high in salt, such as
  – canned soup, dried soup mixes, bouillon
  – canned vegetables and vegetable juices

1. Swelling in the abdomen caused by fluid retention is called "ascites"; when it occurs in the legs, swelling caused by fluid retention is known as "edema."

- cheeses, lower in fat
- margarine
- condiments such as ketchup and soy sauce
- crackers and baked goods
- processed lean meats
- snack foods such as chips, pretzels, and nuts

- Buy fresh vegetables or ones that have been frozen or canned without salt added. Use fresh poultry, fish, and lean meat, rather than canned or processed types.
- Instead of adding salt when cooking, use herbs, spices, and salt-free seasoning blends.
- Don't add salt when cooking rice, pasta, and hot cereals. Avoid buying instant or flavored rice, pasta, and cereal mixes because they usually have added salt.
- Rinse canned foods such as tuna to remove some sodium.
- Choose "convenience" foods that are low in sodium. Cut back on frozen dinners, mixed dishes such as pizza, packaged mixes, canned soups or broth, and salad dressings, which often have a lot of sodium.

The Importance of Getting Enough Fluids

It's especially important for you to drink enough fluids, which will lessen the symptoms of HCV by helping to cleanse your system of toxins. Fluids are important if you are taking interferon, as they reduce side effects. You can calculate how many ounces of liquids you need to drink every day by dividing your body weight in pounds in half. For example, if you are a 180-pound man, you need to consume 90 ounces of liquids—or more than ten 8-ounce glasses of fluid a day. Water is best, but if it makes it more appealing, it's also acceptable to drink juice, seltzer, sports drinks, or milk. Alcoholic beverages should be avoided by anyone with HCV (see page 111–12). Caffeinated drinks can be consumed in moderation, but they should not be factored into your daily quota of fluids consumed, as they actually cause you to lose water. In fact, for every caffeinated drink you should drink an equal-sized glass of water *in addition to* the amount of fluids you are supposed to drink every day.

Vitamin and Mineral Supplements

If you eat a balanced diet, you probably won't need a vitamin or mineral supplement. But if your appetite has been affected and you're not getting enough of the right nutrients, you may indeed need a supplement. Before you take any vitamin or mineral supplement, speak to your doctor. As a general guideline, you should take a supplement that provides no more than one or two times the government's recommended dietary allowance (RDA). If you have HCV, certain substances can cause problems. Some fat-soluble vitamins, such as vitamin A, and some minerals, such as iron, are retained in the liver and may be harmful when taken in large doses.

Overcoming Common Eating Problems Associated with HCV

Both HCV and its drug treatment can cause changes that affect eating patterns. Appetite loss, nausea, and even vomiting are common. People with HCV frequently don't feel like eating. In people with advanced liver disease, such as cirrhosis, significant weight loss can occur. The next section contains practical suggestions for people who have eating problems associated with HCV.

As a general rule, make the most of every mouthful. And even if you can't eat large portions, choose foods high in calories and protein.

If You've Lost Your Appetite

Keep your portions small; a full plate can appear overwhelming. Try exercising a couple of hours before mealtime to stimulate your appetite. Avoid caffeinated drinks (including colas), which are appetite suppressants. Keep plenty of healthy snacks handy, especially foods you like. If it makes you want to eat, don't hesitate to splurge on higher-priced items such as exotic fruit or gourmet crackers. Some people have a larger appetite earlier in the day, so you may want to try to make your morning meal your largest. Indeed, try to get as much as one-third of your total calories at breakfast and use nutritional supplements later in the day when you don't feel like eating.

If Your Senses of Taste and Smell Have Changed

HCV can cause changes in chemical pathways that can alter the way your food tastes. So can interferon, the main medicine used to treat hepatitis C. Certain foods might now taste bitter, especially red meat. Unless you have liver failure, it's important that you eat enough protein, however, as it gives you strength, rebuilds liver cells, and helps you resist infection. If you find red meat tastes unpleasant even though it was previously your principal source of protein, try chicken, fish, or other foods high in protein, such as eggs, peanut butter, beans, cheese, tuna, and yogurt. If you find that hot, just-cooked meat tastes unpleasant, try letting it cool to room temperature. Many people with HCV find that doing so improves the taste. Changes in taste often resolve in time, especially if you're on medication only temporarily. Keep taste-testing foods to see whether they have become palatable again.

Your sense of smell may have changed also. If

you find that food smells offensive to you, try these measures:

- Serve foods at room temperature.
- Open the kitchen window and turn on the kitchen fan when cooking and during the meal.
- Cook outside on a grill when weather permits, or cook in boiling bags or in a microwave oven.
- Use a small fan next to your plate.
- In a hospital setting, ask the person serving the food or a family member to take the lid off your plate before entering your room; if this isn't practical, remove the lid from your food plate away from you.

If You Often Feel Nauseated

Nausea is a common symptom of HCV, and it is one of the most common obstacles to eating well. Even if you have lingering nausea, try not to go for long periods without eating. Eat small portions every two to three hours and eat slowly. Remember, if you are vomiting you need to replace lost fluids (see pages 106–7). Avoid foods that will upset your stomach, such as citrus fruits and juices, which can be hard on the stomach because of their acidity. Better choices are apple or grape juice, chicken or vegetable broth, weak tea, or sports drinks. If you feel especially nauseated in the morning, eat foods that are easy to digest, such as a few dry crackers or bread. Preparing food can make you feel worse, so have prepared food on hand that you can microwave. Medicine to relieve nausea is available, so if it becomes a serious problem, call your doctor.

If You Feel Full Quickly

If you have HCV, your liver may be so inflamed that it may press against your stomach, making you feel full after eating only a small amount or when you've had nothing to eat at all. You can get around this by eating small portions of food up to six times a day, instead of three large meals, and by snacking regularly on healthy foods. The following are some ideas for healthy snacks:

- reduced-fat or fat-free crackers
- air-popped popcorn
- raw vegetables
- rice cakes
- frozen grapes or strawberries
- nonfat frozen yogurt, fat-free ice cream, sorbet, juice bars, or fruit spritzers

Alcohol and Your Liver

Alcohol puts a great strain on your liver and in excessive quantities causes damage to this important organ. Because you already have a disease that affects your liver, you must protect it from any unnecessary further damage. Therefore, avoid alcohol completely or risk the likelihood your disease will worsen rapidly.

Drinking alcohol, in addition to causing unnecessary damage to your liver, will make it difficult for your doctor to determine whether additional liver damage revealed from testing your liver for HCV is the result of your alcohol consumption or the infection in your blood.

Finally, anyone with HCV should avoid alcohol and acetaminophen (an ingredient found in many pain relievers and cold formulas). The two have been linked to a type of liver failure called "fulminant hepatitis," which usually proves fatal.

Unfortunately, for many people—alcoholics in particular—abstaining from alcohol is not a straightforward matter. One characteristic of alcoholism is that alcoholics are unable to control how much they drink—a characteristic which, leaving aside the other problems associated with alcoholism, has potentially lethal consequences for people with HCV.

Regrettably, the emotional and psychological pain caused by a chronic illness such as HCV can provide the impetus for alcoholics to abuse alcohol even more.

If you have HCV and think you might be an active alcoholic, seek help through treatment or by attending a support group. Alcoholics Anonymous has worked for millions of people trying to live one day at a time without taking a drink.

CHAPTER SIX

Liver Transplantation

HCV is the most common reason for needing a liver transplant in the United States today, and the virus is responsible for nearly one-third of all transplants nationally. Liver transplants are the most difficult single-organ transplants—and the most expensive at about $250,000 per procedure. It is important if you have HCV to know under what circumstances you may need a transplant.

The Progression to End-Stage HCV

The liver is an uncomplaining organ; even when it is diseased, it can usually carry on working effectively for a while. Because the liver is so resilient, you may have suffered some HCV-induced liver damage and not know it. But once the damage to your liver becomes severe, the progression from feeling normal to being very ill is quite rapid, and the symptoms can be felt in different organs.

Fluid may accumulate in your abdomen, a condition

known as "ascites," which can interfere with your breathing and may lead to dangerous infections. A condition called "encephalopathy" may develop, in which mental function becomes impaired. This may begin as mild disorientation, progress to drowsiness, and become so serious you go into a coma. Bleeding in your intestinal tract can occur due to increased pressure in the main blood vessel serving your liver, a condition known as "portal hypertension". During the early stages of symptoms, medications can control these symptoms. As liver disease progresses toward its final stages, however, the medications no longer help.

Liver transplantation is the only treatment available for end-stage liver disease. Decisions about if and when to perform the transplant are ones that need to be made by doctors expert in liver disease and liver transplantation. Because it is a nonreversible procedure, it is crucial that only people who will benefit from a transplant have one.

Are You a Transplant Candidate?

When to perform a transplant is a complex issue. If you have HCV, you need to have your condition closely followed by a doctor. If signs of liver damage are detected through a biopsy, you'll probably be referred to a gastroenterologist (a doctor specializing in digestive diseases and liver diseases). Still, it may be many years before you need a transplant—if you ever need one at all.

The final decision for who should or shouldn't have a transplant is usually made by a team of doctors at a liver transplant center. A variety of factors—not a single piece of health information—are taken into consideration. Active alcoholics and drug addicts usually aren't considered.

Following are some of the general criteria that will be used to assess the severity of your liver disease:

- jaundice
- fluid retention
- fatigue
- blood clotting
- indications of portal hypertension
- muscle wasting
- bleeding from the esophagus or stomach

These criteria are evaluated along with the history of your liver disease (how long the symptoms have been present, whether the symptoms are getting worse, and whether the symptoms are due to the liver disease itself), your overall health, and the cause of your liver disease to determine if you should receive a transplant.

As a basic guideline, damage to your liver must be severe enough to make a transplant necessary, but you have to be healthy enough to survive the procedure.

Survival Rates for Transplants

The survival rate among those who have liver transplants is approximately 80 percent at one year and 70 percent at five years. There are no firm statistics on how long a transplanted liver will last. Twenty-five years is the longest recorded survival for a liver transplant patient. Ten-year survival is common. New surgery techniques and medications to prevent rejection of the transplanted liver are expected to improve survival rates, as well as improve the quality of life for transplant patients.

Will a Transplant Cure Your HCV?

Unfortunately, a liver transplant is no cure if you have HCV. That's because the virus lives in cells in other parts of your body. Once the new liver is connected, the virus will spread to it within a few weeks. No treatment is available to prevent this from happening. While the majority of patients don't have serious effects from re-infection, the virus causes serious liver damage in about 20 percent of transplants. Five percent experience liver failure within three to five years. Retransplantation fails in more than 50 percent of cases.

Waiting Time for a Liver

The waiting time for a liver doubled between 1991 and 1996 to 241 days. And, given the large number of people with HCV, this situation will almost certainly worsen over the next few years. In the United States, it is soon expected that 50 percent of hopeful recipients will die waiting for a liver.

With transplantable livers in short supply relative to the increased demand, a solution for HCV patients in desperate circumstances has been to give them organs that others don't want. In particular, livers from donors who are also HCV-infected. A biopsy is done of the donor liver, and if it shows only mild damage, it may be used. The liver may be from a donor who recovered and whose liver showed only leftover antibodies to HCV or may even have been a false-positive. No matter what, a successful transplant extends life.

The Procedure

The most common type of liver transplant is an "orthotopic" liver transplant. It involves three separate procedures:

- removal of the recipient's liver
- removal of the donor's liver
- implantation of the donor liver into the recipient

Removing the recipient's liver, is the most difficult of the three procedures. There are several reasons why:

- The liver makes the substances in the blood that cause clotting. Diseased livers don't make enough of these substances; therefore, HCV-positive patients have a tendency to bleed excessively during surgery.

- Portal hypertension, a condition that causes the blood to get congested as the liver tries to filter it, is common in people with diseased livers and makes the procedure more difficult.

- Many people who need a liver transplant have cirrhosis, a scarring process that makes the liver more difficult to separate from adjoining tissues.

The donor's liver is usually removed at the hospital where the person died, except when there is a brain-dead "living donor," in which case the donor is in the operating room beside the recipient. The procedure is usually not complicated. The removed liver is cooled, the blood is flushed out of it, and a preservative solution is flushed in. Then it is kept in a plastic bag over ice until it is ready to be transplanted into the donor.

With the recipient under general anesthesia, an incision is made under the ribs. The abdominal muscles are separated or split, and the peritoneal cavity is opened. The liver and its bile ducts are isolated and then cut free and removed. With the recipient's old liver out, the donor liver is inserted by connecting the blood vessels and bile ducts. When blood flow to the organ resumes, the liver should start making blood-clotting substances and the portal hypertension should go away. The peritoneum and abdominal muscles are closed, the incision stitched shut, and the transplant is completed.

Often bleeding continues for several hours or days after the surgery, even when the procedure goes exactly as planned. The liver, because it was on ice for some time, may be working sluggishly. In about one out of five cases doctors have to perform a second procedure to remove accumulated blood.

Early Recovery

Recovery time depends on how ill you were prior to the surgery. You should count on spending a few days in the intensive care unit (ICU) and a minimum of about three weeks in the hospital ward.

During the period in the ICU, doctors will carefully monitor all your body functions, especially those of your liver. When you are transferred to the ward, the frequency of the blood testing and other evaluations will be decreased, eating is permitted, and physical therapy is started so you will regain muscle strength. At this stage the drugs used to prevent rejection of the new liver are given intraveneously (into the vein), then later orally (by mouth).

Post-surgery Treatment

One of the most important components of treatment after surgery is drugs to prevent rejection of your new liver. These are known as "immunosuppressive medicines." Unfortunately, these drugs increase your susceptibility to infections. Several different medicines are used, and each causes its own problems. Cortisone-like drugs cause fluid retention and puffiness in the face, increase the risk of worsening diabetes, and may speed up the process of osteoporosis (a bone-thinning condition). Cyclosporine is associated with increased blood pressure and kidney damage, and so dosages of this medicine must be carefully regulated (it is also linked to growth of body hair). Common side effects of a drug called FK-506 are headaches, tremor, diarrhea, anxiety, nausea, and kidney dysfunction.

Usually, recipients of liver transplants must take these medications for the rest of their lives; however, as the body adjusts to the new liver, dosages of the medicines can be reduced. Some patients have been weaned off the drugs completely. Doctors are trying to determine why some patients are able to live with their new liver without the need for immunosuppressive drugs.

Routine follow-up consists of monthly blood tests, blood pressure tests by your family physician, and annual or semiannual checkups at the transplant center.

As the immune system is usually affected by the drugs prescribed to prevent your body from rejecting your new liver, it is important to avoid exposure to viruses and bacteria. Any illness should be reported immediately to your doctor, and medicines for the infection should be taken only under medical supervision.

Diet, Exercise, and Recreation

After a successful transplant, most patients can return to normal or near-normal existence and can participate in fairly strenuous exercise six to twelve months after the procedure. Refer to pages 85–89 for information on a walking program for beginners. As with other activities, sexual activity may be resumed soon after getting out of the hospital, as long as commonsense precautions are observed.

Transplant patients have a tendency to retain water. For this reason, they should avoid salty foods to reduce or eliminate fluid retention. Otherwise you should maintain a balanced diet. For more information on a suitable diet, refer to pages 103–6.

Although liver failure may occur after transplantation, and even when it doesn't, there is the possibility that your HCV will strike against your new liver. Regardless, if you undergo a liver transplant, the odds are in your favor that you will survive the procedure and go on to live a healthy, productive life with your new organ. And as medical technology continues to improve, the survival rates will too.

About Organ Donation

Livers are received, with consent of the next of kin, from people who have been rendered brain dead, usually as a result of a massive head injury. When such a donor is identified, transplant centers are notified via computer and arrangements are made to retrieve whatever organs may be donated. Often this necessitates a team from a transplant center flying to the donor hospital to remove the organs and returning with them for the transplant operations.

The donor and recipient do not have to be matched by tissue type, sex, age, and so forth. For liver transplants, the only requirements are that the donor and recipient need to be approximately the same size and of compatible blood types. No other matching is necessary.

If there are two suitable recipients for a donated liver—not a common occurrence—the patient whose need is more urgent usually receives the liver.

Someone who has HCV is not usually eligible to donate his or her liver, except in certain cases (see page 117). You can urge family and friends to be donors. If someone you know wishes to be an organ donor, he or she needs to carry an organ donor card and place an organ donor sticker on his or her medical identification card. It is important that organ donors discuss the subject with family members, as they will have to give consent. An organ donor card is available from the American Liver Foundation.

CHAPTER SEVEN

Complementary and Alternative Treatments for HCV

You have turned over control of your disease to a Higher Power. In doing so you have agreed to do your part in taking care of yourself. That includes finding out what treatments are available that may help alleviate or improve your condition, even those treatments outside the realm of conventional medicine.

Complementary and alternative medicines are treatments and health care approaches not taught widely in Western medical schools, not generally used in hospitals, and not usually reimbursed by medical insurance. The terms cover a wide range of ancient healing philosophies, approaches, and therapies.

The terms "alternative" and "complementary" are not interchangeable. Therapies used *instead of* conventional medicine are considered to be alternative. Therapies used *in conjunction with* conventional medicine are referred to as complementary.

Certain complementary and alternative approaches are based on familiar principles of Western medicine, but many have quite different origins. Many therapies remain far outside the realm of accepted Western medicine, while others have been embraced by large segments of society.

Consider, for instance, the ancient Chinese medical practice of acupuncture. Once considered quite bizarre in the West, it is now increasingly used by ordinary Americans to treat common medical conditions, to relieve stress, and even to ease symptoms during nicotine withdrawal. The same is true for herbal medicine, as evidenced by the television commercials for products containing echinacea, ginseng, and Saint-John's-wort. Given their increasing popularity among those attracted by low cost, lack of side effects, and purported effectiveness, many forms of medicine presently considered offbeat will eventually become accepted by mainstream health culture.

It is a measure of society's interest in alternatives to conventional medicine that in 1992 the government-run National Institutes of Health (NIH) created an Office of Alternative Medicine (OAM). The OAM facilitates research and evaluation of unconventional medical practices and disseminates this information to the public. Its budget in 1998 was $20 million. You can obtain a classification of forty-seven complementary and alternative medical health care practices from the OAM. The list is intended to show the diversity of the field and is neither complete nor authoritative.

Many practitioners of conventional health care continue to dispute the claims of alternative and complementary medicine. That is because, by and large, such therapies are not investigated using the same scientific research methods used in conventional medicine. The benefits of such treatments, Western-trained doctors argue, is strictly anecdotal; that is, based on patient testimonials not documented results. It is unlikely that alternative and complementary medicine will be fully accepted until its practitioners can produce results based on rigorous research methods dependent upon systematic, explicit, and comprehensive knowledge and skills.

How to Find Out More about Complementary and Alternative Treatments for HCV

Health care providers are becoming more familiar with alternative and complementary treatments, and your doctor may be willing to refer you to such a practitioner. The medical profession, however, is by and large suspicious of medical treatments it considers untested, unproven, and thus potentially harmful.

Don't be discouraged if your doctor cannot or will not provide you with the information you want. Information about particular complementary and alternative medical practices is available on the Internet, in medical libraries, in public libraries, and in popular bookstores.

Other resources for alternative and complementary therapies are the NIH's twenty-four institutes, centers, and divisions. For information from the NIH on HCV, call (301) 496-4000 and ask the operator to direct you to the appropriate office.

If you are online, access to most medical research resources on the Internet is free. Some sites—such as www.thriveonline.com—take the latest medical research and translate it into information the ordinary person can understand. An excellent online source of complementary and alternative medicine is the alternative medicine section of www.healthanswers.com. Lessons in the basics of using the Internet are widely available, and classes may be held at your local library, senior center, or adult learning center.

To find out more about complementary and alternative treatments for hepatitis C, you may also want to ask practitioners of complementary and alternative medicine about their practices. Many practitioners belong to professional associations, educational organizations, and research institutions that provide information about complementary and alternative medical practices. A growing number of these organizations have sites on the Internet.

Be aware that some organizations advocate a specific therapy or treatment but are unable to provide complete and objective health information. Before trying out any treatment, get as much information as you can and discuss your findings and thoughts with your doctor.

How to Find a Practitioner in Your Area

To find a qualified complementary or alternative medical health care practitioner, contact medical regulatory and licensing agencies in your state (your health care provider should be able to provide you with their names). Such regulatory and licensing bodies can provide information about a specific practitioner's credentials and background. Many states license practitioners who provide alternative therapies such as acupuncture, chiropractic services, and massage therapy.

You also may locate individual practitioners by asking your health care provider or by contacting a professional association or organization. These organizations can provide names of local practitioners and information about how to determine the quality of a specific practitioner's services.

Choosing an Alternative Health Care Therapy or Practitioner

The health decisions you make are important, and choosing to explore complementary and alternative treatments is no exception. There are some serious issues you need to address when selecting an alternative or complementary therapy or practitioner. In particular, ask questions about the safety and effectiveness of the treatment, the qualifications of the practitioner, and the cost of the therapy.

Is It Safe? Is It Effective?

The therapy should provide relief from the condition for which it is sought—in this case, HCV—and it should not have the ability to cause you harm when used as intended. Unfortunately, less is known about the safety and effectiveness of complementary and alternative products and practices than conventional medicine. So what can you do?

Ask the health practitioner for evidence of the safety and effectiveness of the practice, treatment, or technology he or she advocates. Request information on new research that either supports or debunks the effectiveness of the treatment, and also ask about any new information about its safety.

You should also ask questions about possible side effects, interactions with other medications you are taking, expected results, and how long the treatment should last.

Make sure the practitioner is aware of all other therapies—both conventional and alternative or complementary—you are using, as this information will probably be necessary to ensure the safety and effectiveness of the treatment plan.

Published information on the safety and effectiveness of particular therapies can be found in scientific journals available at certain public libraries, university libraries, medical libraries, online computer services, and the U.S. National Library of Medicine (NLM) at the National Institutes of Health. As the articles in these journals can be difficult for the layperson to understand, you might find the summary at the beginning of the manuscript, known as the "abstract," the easiest way to gain information from these materials. You can find these scientific articles in the *Index Medicus,* a published resource available in medical and university libraries and some public libraries.

The World Wide Web can be an excellent source of information about the safety and effectiveness of complementary and alternative medicine, although it is important that you learn to differentiate between credible and noncredible sources. This ability to discern comes in part with time spent using the Internet.

Also, try to gain access to people with HCV who have received the treatment you are researching. Remember, though, that anecdotal evidence from other patients is not an accurate measure of the safety and effectiveness of a treatment. It should not be the sole criteria for selecting an alternative or complementary therapy. Studies done under controlled conditions by trained medical scientists are the best way to assess a treatment's effectiveness.

What Are the Practitioner's Qualifications?

Research the background, qualifications, and reputation of the practitioner. You can do this by contacting the state or local regulatory body that has jurisdiction over the practice of the therapy you are seeking. Although complementary and alternative medicine is not as strictly regulated as conventional medicine, licensing and accreditation are continually being introduced.

Local and state medical boards may be able to provide information about an individual practitioner's credentials, and consumer affairs departments such as the Better Business Bureau can tell you whether there have been any complaints lodged against that person.

How Much Does It Cost?

Your health insurer or the practitioner should be able to tell you whether a particular therapy is covered by insurance; however, most complementary and alternative treatments are not covered by health insurance. Patients usually have to pay the entire amount of the therapy. Thus, cost is an important factor for people seeking alternative and complementary medical treatment.

Shop around to find out what different practitioners charge for the same service. Although cost shouldn't be the sole criteria for selection, knowing what a variety of practitioners charge will give you some idea of what is appropriate. The same professional and regulatory bodies that can provide information on safety and effectiveness should be able to provide approximate cost guidelines.

Specific Complementary and Alternative Treatments for HCV

Most of the alternative and complementary treatments for HCV involve herbal and nutritional supplements as well as nutritional therapy. Some people with HCV claim without reservation that they have been able to improve their condition using herbs. Others have found that herbs do no good at all in relieving their symptoms or slowing the progression of their HCV. Where does the truth lie? No one really knows without controlled studies. It's up to you as an individual to decide whether or not you should use herbal remedies for your condition.

First, you should know certain facts.

Above all, it is important to never take certain herbs or megadose vitamins that are "hepatoxic" (harmful to your liver). Herbs known to destroy liver cells and tissue and that should *NOT* be taken if you have HCV include

- comfrey (bush tea)
- germander
- chaparral
- Jin Bu Huan
- nutmeg
- pennyroyal
- mistletoe
- tansy
- ragwort
- senna
- sassafras
- valerian

In those with HCV, ingesting these herbs has been associated with conditions ranging from acute hepatitis and jaundice to cirrhosis and death from liver failure.

On the other hand, certain natural substances have been proved to be beneficial for people with HCV. The most effective herbal treatment is from the berries of the plant milk thistle, which contain a chemical called "silymarin." Milk thistle has been found in some studies to stimulate the regeneration of liver cells and to protect liver cells not already damaged by the virus. Significantly, milk thistle has not been shown to have any harmful side effects. German health authorities have approved milk thistle as a treatment for HCV. Milk thistle is *not* a cure for HCV and does not work against liver cancer.

Milk thistle can be taken in capsule or alcohol-free extract form. Recommended dosage is 200 to 400 milligrams three times daily. It can be bought over the counter in most drugstores.

Whether or not to use herbal treatments is a personal choice. Above all, it is essential to keep your doctor informed about all the medicines you are taking, herbs included.

Appendix

The following organizations provide extensive information about HCV and other liver diseases.

Hepatitis C Foundation
National Headquarters
1502 Russett Drive
Warminster, PA 18974
Telephone: (215) 672-2606
Fax: (215) 672-1518
E-mail: hepc@hepcfoundation.org

Hepatitis Foundation International
30 Sunrise Terrace
Cedar Grove, NJ 07009-1423
Internet site: www.hepfi.org
Telephone: (800) 891-0707
Fax: (973) 857-5044
E-mail: mail@hepfi.org

Centers for Disease Control and Prevention—
  Hepatitis Branch
1600 Clifton Road
Atlanta, GA 30333
Internet site: www.cdc.gov/ncidod/diseases/
  hepatitis/hepatitis.htm
Telephone: (888) 4HEPCDC or (888) 443-7232

American Liver Foundation
75 Maiden Lane, Suite 603
New York, NY 10038
Internet site: www.liverfoundation.org
Telephone: (800) 465-4837 or (800) GOLIVER
E-mail: webmail@liverfoundation.org

American Association for the Study of Liver Diseases
1729 King Street, Suite 1000
Alexandria, VA 22314-2720
Internet site: www.aasld.org
Telephone: (703) 299-9766
Fax: (703) 299-9622
E-mail: aasld@aasld.org

Canadian Liver Foundation
National Office
365 Bloor Street East, Suite 200
Toronto, Ontario M4W 3L4
Internet site: www.liver.ca
Telephone: (416) 964-1953
Toll-free: (800) 563-5483
Fax: (416) 964-0024
E-mail: clf@liver.ca

Index

About the Author

MARK JENKINS is the author of several books on health. He co-wrote *The Sports Medicine Bible,* a Book-of-the-Month Club alternate selection. Jenkins lives year-round on the island of Martha's Vineyard off the coast of Cape Cod, Massachusetts. He travels occasionally to the mainland by ferryboat to fulfill his duties as publishing consultant at the world-renowned Boston Children's Hospital.

HAZELDEN INFORMATION AND EDUCATIONAL SERVICES is a division of the Hazelden Foundation, a not-for-profit organization. Since 1949, Hazelden has been a leader in promoting the dignity and treatment of people afflicted with the disease of chemical dependency.

The mission of the foundation is to improve the quality of life for individuals, families, and communities by providing a national continuum of information, education, and recovery services that are widely accessible; to advance the field through research and training; and to improve our quality and effectiveness through continuous improvement and innovation.

Stemming from that, the mission of this division is to provide quality information and support to people wherever they may be in their personal journey—from education and early intervention, through treatment and recovery, to personal and spiritual growth.

Although our treatment programs do not necessarily use everything Hazelden publishes, our bibliotherapeutic materials support our mission and the Twelve Step philosophy upon which it is based. We encourage your comments and feedback.

The headquarters of the Hazelden Foundation is in Center City, Minnesota. Additional treatment facilities are located in Chicago, Illinois; New York, New York; Plymouth, Minnesota; St. Paul, Minnesota; and West Palm Beach, Florida. At these sites, we provide a continuum of care for men and women of all ages. Our Plymouth facility is designed specifically for youth and families.

For more information on Hazelden, please call **1-800-257-7800.** Or you may access our World Wide Web site on the Internet at **www.hazelden.org.**